AUTOIMMUNITY
COUNTER-ATTACK

"A major women's health issue…"
National Institute of Health's Office of Research on Women's Health

AWARENESS FUND-RAISER:

BICYCLING COAST-TO-COAST

ANONYMOUS GG

ISBN 0-7414-1792-8

DISCLAIMER

This book was written for the purposes of health education awareness regarding autoimmunity and hypersensitivity. The contents herein should not be used as a substitute for medical care. Please consult your qualified medical doctor(s) and support organizations for your healthcare needs.

Published by:

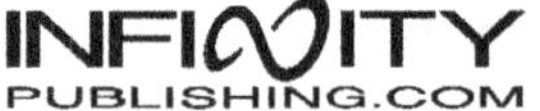

519 West Lancaster Avenue
Haverford, PA 19041-1413
Info@buybooksontheweb.com
www.buybooksontheweb.com
Toll-free (877) BUY BOOK
Local Phone (610) 520-2500
Fax (610) 519-0261

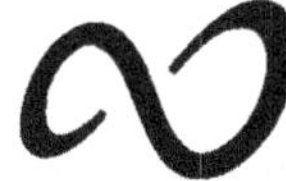

Printed in the United States of America

Printed on Recycled Paper

Published November 2003

AUTHOR'S NOTE

Some names within are fictitious. The story and facts are real. Fifty percent of author's profits will be donated to the American Autoimmune Related Disease Association, a non-profit organization dedicated to health education regarding autoimmunity as an etiology of disease. Increased understanding, early diagnosis, adequate medical intervention, efficient management, and, ideally, eradication of autoimmune related diseases are the goals of AARDA and this book.

Twenty-five percent of author's profits will be donated to The Lupus Foundation of America, Northwest, Indiana Chapter. Twelve percent will be donated to The Multiple Sclerosis Society. The remaining 13% will be directed toward a Fibromyalgia organization, Northwest, Indiana Chapter and The Arthritis Foundation, South Bend, Indiana Chapter, for use regarding Juvenile Rheumatoid Arthritis.

Come ride along as we all journey away from mis-understanding, disability and death. Celebrate our ascension toward prevention, healthy management, and the wonders of wellness.

(NOTE: Any formatting variations are due to the author, since there was no time to send this disk back into NerdWorld again.)

Best Wishes for Optimal Health!
Author, Anonymous GG, L.P.N.
B.A. Health and Wellness Education
Hyper-Immune System and Chronic
Pain Survivor

FOR ALL OF US AND IN HONOR OF THE BRAVE,
RESILIENT FIGHTING SPIRIT.

ACKNOWLEDGMENTS

I owe it all to Holly and Sissy. My beloved canine kids gave me a family to come home to and provided love, laughter, and company during the sickest of times. (Thanks to their entrusted doggy-sitters too!)

Much gratitude to a kind-hearted lady named Marge. During the toughest of times, you made sure I remained in the comforts of my home.

To my family and friends. You know how much you mean to me. Thanks always for being there.

To that neat pastor who entered my life when needed and church full of friendly, welcoming folks. You helped!

To all of my dedicated employers, fellow working class comrades, and inspiring people I served, you helped too!

To my guardian angels who guided me every step of the way. What a remarkable enlightening journey! As always, I'm forever in your debt and I hope this book is all you meant it to be. Don't forget to visit.

Once again, I must thank technology because without the Internet, many links may not have connected so quickly or cohesively. So here's a toast to the Internet and all of the resources utilized. "Job well done!"

To my aides: bronchodilators, antihistamines, immuno-suppressive and anti-inflammatory medications. No words could ever express how grateful I am for those precious gifts, counteraction and quality of life. The same goes to Henry, my imaginary friend, that enlightened, protective antibody rescuer. It was all possible because of you! And you too, my fine, caring, exceptional doctor, thank God you didn't retire!

To all other valiant warriors, personally or professionally caught up in the immunological wars, fight on, we need you!

For our dear fallen soldiers, you are not forgotten.

Notice to my Adventure Cycling Tour guide and coast to coast bicycling pals, I'm counting on you to see me through! Happy, healthy traveling days, always!

To Vivian at Nerd World Productions in New York, my phenomenal literary assistant, what a miracle worker!

CONTENTS

INTRODUCTION

Someday there will be a cure for multiple sclerosis, rheumatoid arthritis, Grave's disease, type I immune-mediated diabetes, strange-sounding afflictions named systemic lupus erythematosus and thrombocytopenic purpura, and many other autoimmune related diseases. Scientists, researchers, healthcare professionals, and many organizations are working diligently to understand the causes and adverse effects of autoimmunity while enabling those afflicted to enjoy an improved quality of life. Health education, prevention, healthy management, and especially eradication of disease, disability, and death are the goals.

Yet, unlike cancer which is a well-known category or etiology of disease, autoimmunity which is responsible for the underlying cause of at least 80 chronic illnesses, remains "among the most poorly understood and poorly recognized of any category of illness." (1) The diseases are often referred to by using lengthy, barely able to pronounce, confusing names. Millions suffer from autoimmunity, yet when asked what the name of their disease is, sometimes it's very difficult to get the words right, let alone explain how the disease process works. Imagine trying to ramble off a diagnosis of ankylosing spondylitis, myasthenis gravis, Hashimoto's thyroiditis, antiphospholid antibody syndrome, or systemic lupus erythematosus or a histio(tissue) *in*compatibility of some sort and expect someone to understand what disease is causing so much misery and threat to quality of life, or life.

Autoimmune related diseases rank high on the priority list of the National Institute of Health, Office of Research on Women's Health. Some fifty million Americans are afflicted and autoimmunity targets women 75% of the time. Autoimmunity represents the 4th largest cause of disease among women in the U.S., and one study reported that autoimmune diseases made the top ten list of leading causes of all deaths among U.S. women, 65 and younger. (2)

So what is autoimmunity exactly? What is this disease process that is causing so much disability and death? Well, let me introduce you and hopefully increase your understanding of autoimmunity, as an etiology of disease, if you are not aware of it.

I've thought about this quite a bit and I think the easiest way to explain autoimmunity, for people who are just learning about autoimmune diseases or for someone who wants to gain a better understanding, is to refer first to the immunization process. Most people understand immunizations, vaccines, at least somewhat, right?

The reason why many life-threatening illnesses no longer pose a threat to the human race is because immunization provides a strong defense against deadly diseases. "Vaccines contain a weakened (attenuated) or killed (inactivated) form of disease-causing bacteria or viruses, or components of these microorganisms, that trigger a response by our body's immune system."(3) Talk about adaptation. We need protection from a deadly disease and all we have to do is introduce a little bit of the weakened or dead form of it into our systems and our body sees it as an enemy, attacks and destroys. "Vaccines stimulate our bodies to make antibodies-proteins that specifically recognize and target the bacteria and viruses against which the vaccines are designed, and that helps eliminate them from the body when we encounter them."(4)

Unfortunately, there are always new bacterial and viral diseases emerging, and it can take years to develop a safe, effective vaccine. If it were a simple process, many infectious diseases, AIDS (acquired immune deficiency disease syndrome), and even the multitude of immuno-logically-caused illnesses might no longer be a threat to us.

In the case of immunization and allergies, the immune system reacts, hurries to our defense. An invader threatens us, then our body, equipped with antibodies to the invasive substance, counterattacks. Allergic individuals, unfor-tunately, must deal with hypersensitive immune systems, and far too often the immune system reacts to harmless substances, for example: dust, pollen, or certain foods such as peanuts or shrimp.

"The disease-producing mechanisms in autoimmunity are called hypersensitivity reactions. These reactions also occur in allergies, which are related phenomena. Both are inappropriate responses of the immune system except that, with allergy, the response is to invading substances (antigens) from outside the body."(5)

Autoimmunity occurs "when there is some interruption of the usual control process, allowing lympho-cytes to avoid suppression, or when there is an alteration of some body tissue so that it is no longer recognized as self and is thus attacked."(6) This can be disastrous for a person who is afflicted with an autoimmune related disease.

There are so many different names for autoimmune diseases. Rather than eighty or more various, difficult to pronounce and spell, disease names; like cancer or allergies, as autoimmunity is better understood as an etiology of disease, a person could simply say, "I have an autoimmune problem or illness," or "I suffer from autoimmunity." Where the cancer activity is denotes a specific site for cancer. Where the allergic or autoimmune reaction occurs, that may describe the location better, but the cause of an autoimmune disease is still autoimmunity.

"The common thread" in all of the autoimmune related diseases, as Dr. Neil Rose, advisor for AARDA, would say is of course, autoimmunity. This is what's important to understand. "The common etiology that brings together all of these diseases is autoimmunity." (7)

Defining diseases by what causes the problem and developing action plans to counterattack the underlying reasons for a disease process, rather than simply treating the symptoms after the fact makes much more sense. Yet to prevent something from occurring, the cause of the problem must first be the primary concern. We already know in the case of cancer, often the symptoms show up later, after the disease has been present for quite some time. Cancer treatment exists, but early detection is crucial and understanding and counteracting the cause of illness is imperative, not merely trying to fight the symptoms and allowing the essential trigger(s) of disease to continue.

Although, for some diseases unfortunately, after a certain amount of damage is done, and for some conditions, management of inevitable symptoms, rather than prevention or a cure, is sometimes the only option. Quality of life is often obtained with health education and proper management of a disease. However, it still always helps to understand what causes a particular disease and symptoms, even if irreversible. And it's that understanding of the etiology of a disease which still offers the best chance for researchers to make progress toward preventive measures and cures.

The fact that anti-inflammatory and immuno-suppressive medications work to counteract or suppress the symptoms of autoimmunity and/or prevent damage means that if someone knows that autoimmunity is causing the problems, help is on the way. PERMANENT damage can be prevented! LIVES CAN BE SAVED! There is great potential for preventive medicine and preservation of quality of life, even life, with relation to autoimmune related diseases. It's time to COUNTERATTACK, even prevent, the devastating effects of autoimmunity. With increased awareness, positive solutions, effective healthcare, and tremendous humanitarian support will follow.

For those of us who fight the immunological wars within, we have already resolved to counterattack. We may be wounded, and at times we are sick. But as Montel Williams professes, "WE ARE NOT WEAK!" We will not give up. We need soldier companions. Let us all work together against the terrorist attacks caused by inner immune-mediated wars responsible for so many related disabilities and casualties.

If auto (self) attack exists, then we can be certain that auto (self) counterattack is possible too. COUNTER-ATTACK! Let's make it a reality. Wars are tough, but we can win, now that we understand the enemy. Remember too, even with casualties of the past, present, or future; we always win, if we do not forget those who fought so bravely before us, and we never surrender our hopeful spirit.

CHAPTER ONE

Mysterious Malady or
Anatomy of a Hypersensitive and/or
Autoimmune Disease?

"All the magnificence of our immune system can be turned against the body and cause disease. It now appears that those early whisperers were right. The immune system, always the counterattacker, sometimes it misreads the signs and launches itself at our cells just as relentlessly as it would any foreign invader."(8)

The Body is the Hero
Dr. Ronald J. Glasser
Bantam Books, 1979, p.79.

"Antibody soldiers patrol, defend, and protect human bodies. When well-intended (but misguided) or rebel over-reactive antibodies terrorize and cause an immune system to become a person's own worst enemy; all one can do is hope, pray, and counterattack."

Autoimmunity Counterattack
Anonymous GG, Author

There once lived a beautiful two year old boy named Ricky. He died. There once lived a happy, seemingly healthy sixteen year old named Amy. She died too. There once lived a young woman of eighteen years named Angel with all of her dreams: attending college, falling in love someday, raising a family and enjoying a career. None of that happened, because, as her life as an adult was just beginning, she also, instead died.

There once lived a beautiful, courageous woman named, Andrea Krane. I wish I could have known her. She tenaciously fought autoimmunity for years. Andrea celebrated life by educating and helping others. She fought relentless inner immunological battles until her last breath. Sadly though, eventually, she too died of a progressive autoimmune related disease process, which took her life.

How many children and adults are we losing to either disability and/or death each day? How many each year, because of autoimmunity? How many autoimmune disease afflicted individuals fail to receive the proper expedient medical intervention, support and understanding that they need?

I visited my dear friend Anne yesterday. You'd love Anne if you knew her. She's about the closest thing to a real live modern day Helen Keller. Just like Helen Keller, one of my beloved heroines, Anne doesn't pay a bit of attention to her limitations. No, she calmly lives out each day, each and every moment, maximizing whatever capabilities she still is lucky enough to hang onto. And what those capabilities exist of since Anne is a multiple sclerosis survivor, is this: her beautiful, loving and highly intelligent mind, the ability to move her head left and right, and thank God her continuous ability to swallow food and drink liquids without choking, and use her mouth and lips to speak. So lucky me, and her family and friends; we still enjoy the wonderful privilege of hearing Anne talk to us.

Attacked and betrayed by her very own immune system, my friend has endured decades of disability and the loss of one precious thing after another because something within her body went haywire. Symptoms began shortly after she received a bite from some sort of guilty culprit. Spider bite or something else, she remains uncertain, but she does remember a red mark, inflammation and pain, and thinks it was either a spider or some other type of bug that bit her leg.

So often our immune system protects, saves us from disease or harm. Tragically though, rather than prevent disease, defend, protect, assist and promote healing, our human complex immune system can quickly act as a villain, a vicious attacker that seeks and destroys, none other than, the cells, tissues, muscles, and/or organs of a person's own body.

There is no disputing it. As Americans, we do not have to travel far away to witness the evils and destruction of war. There's a senseless plague of a war going on right here on American soil, inside human body battlefields. I emphasize senseless, because the war within is indeed often preventable or manageable. When war breaks out within hypersensitive individuals, it happens for one or two reasons: self-defense because actual or perceived foreign invaders have broken through the barriers and need to be destroyed or because of a misguided self-attack. Mistaken as the enemy, the counterattack mechanisms of the immune system target various areas of a victim's own body. Inflammation then occurs, wherever and whenever the body is under attack.

"The term autoimmune disease refers to a varied group of illnesses that involve almost every organ system. It includes disease of the nervous, gastrointestinal, endocrine systems, as well as the skin and other connective tissues, eyes, blood, and blood vessels, including the musculoskeletal system. In all of these diseases, the underlying problem is similar. The body's immune system becomes misdirected, attacks the very organs it was designed to protect." (9)

To answer my earlier question, how many people are afflicted? Approximately fifty million Americans live with autoimmunity. One in five Americans or 20% of the population has an autoimmune disease and approximately 75% of those afflicted are women. (10)

Rheumatoid arthritis, the most crippling form, which is immune-mediated, affects approximately 2.1 million Americans and contributes to major heartache, disability, and incredible loss of productivity. Juvenile rheumatoid arthritis occurs in 70,000 to 75,000 children in the U.S. (11)

Another autoimmune disease, multiple sclerosis, affects approximately 400,000 adult Americans. (stats vary) Experts estimate that 20,000 children have the disease but are undiagnosed. Lauren Krupp, a neurologist at the State University of New York at Stony Brook says, "Misdiagnosing children with MS didn't matter much 10 years ago, when there was no treatment for the disease. Today, an early diagnosis matters a great deal: Neurologists have a number of powerful new drugs at their disposal that can slow the potentially disabling disease." (12)

It is estimated that 500,000 to 1.5 million Americans, again a high proportion are women, have lupus. Lupus, the systemic type, can be severely disabling and/or life-threatening. Sixteen thousand Americans develop lupus every year. (13) Sadly, these devastating statistics only represent part of the overwhelming problem. There is a long list of autoimmune related diseases.

In August of 2001, when my fingers, joints, and wrists began to suddenly swell, stiffen up, and cause excruciating pain and disability; I knew immediately that something was terribly wrong. My first thought of course, since I happened to be at work, went something like, how on earth am I going to function like this? How will I continue to work? I can't even push the medications out. One essential duty of a nurse is to pass the pills that residents are prescribed by their doctors.

Caught off guard and suddenly becoming some type of statistic and experiencing a health crisis nightmare, while agonizing, my body and mind spiraled into a flight for life mode, and hopeful return to a functioning level. Well, things happened. And I have to say at this point, call it what you will, but it seemed that each post-disease step I took thereafter was meant to be, and guided. Yes guided, as if a guardian angel came straight down from heaven, held on tightly to my aching hand, and led me to one answer after another.

The first? It occurred at Burger King in Monticello, Indiana, shortly after my symptoms began. After ordering my usual, a Kid's Meal, plain hamburger, French fries and a Coke; I ruffled through the stack of newspapers on hand and an article stuck out like a red alert medical bracelet. Tina Wesson, a "Survivor" show winner apparently had survived a real life crisis called rheumatoid arthritis. While reading the article as fast as I could race my eyes to the very end, I began to cry. And I said thanks to you know who, because the article was a finger/hand/wrist life-saving gift. I looked down at my temporarily deformed, swollen red right hand and felt so lucky, because I knew I could save it. With antihistamines and thanks to prednisone, I knew I could counterattack, that the horrible signs and symptoms and pain were reversible. Just like other critical or bothersome times in my life due to a hypersensitivity, I could bring my out of control immune system back into a healthy balance and return to normal. I thanked Tina Wesson and that reporter from the bottom of my heart.

A few days after that incident, I got real lucky again. As I sat down at the nurses' station trying to make a dent in the hours of paperwork ahead of me, I looked over to the left and saw a picture of Kellie Martin (the actress), on the cover of Reader's Digest. I began to read all about how her sister, sadly, had died of an autoimmune disease called lupus. It surprised me, for a couple of reasons.

One. I had just returned from a writers' workshop in Muncie, Indiana. As a part-time writer, I attended the event for literary inspirational reasons, but also as a journalist/writer covering a story in order to collect some interviews and insight for a book I was in the midst of writing titled *Author Unknown, Author Undaunted*, regarding the revolutionized publishing industry. My very first interviewee just happened to be Ken Wales, Hollywood producer of the Christy television series. So the name/person of Kellie Martin had just previously popped into my life. I thought, gee, that's a coincidence. I copied the article. Naturally, I got more and more behind in my paperwork as I read the article again, for a second time. Tears again, for Kellie Martin, her sister, Heather, who didn't make it, and her whole family. (Funny how that Reader's Digest was there just long enough for me to see it and copy the article. When I jumped up to go administer a requested medication, I came back and it was gone.)

I felt lucky again too, thanks to the story, just in case I had something more serious than arthritis, I decided I'd be careful and stay one step ahead of any life-threatening damage. I figured joint inflammation is one thing, attack of vital organs quite another, a much more serious condition to make sure I avoided. I spent the next couple of days researching arthritis and lupus. I wanted to learn all I could and prepare to counterattack. Also, if prevention could avoid permanent damage, I knew I had to warn others.

With those first attacks, I was suddenly a disabled person. I thought, forget about working in a nursing home, I may as well just check myself in and let my friends take care of me too. Without the use of my hands, I couldn't even dress myself or brush my hair without excruciating pain. I wondered, do people without these problems have any idea how difficult it is to turn a doorknob, open up a seemingly forever sealed bottle of medication or can of dog food, maneuver a steering wheel, open and shut heavy house windows, or simply carry on when these attacks occur?

Getting tangled up in a sports bra isn't my idea of a humorous situation. Sometimes though, it was either laugh or cry more tears. Due to fear upon movement, it took me a while to get brave and move those painful fingers again to get fully dressed. I slept upstairs. Good thing a rail was there to hold onto. You should have seen the way I had to hobble around the house when other parts of my body acted up, including my feet.

Things got a little better as I acquired knowledge regarding my new assumed "Arthur" nemesis, and adaptive techniques of cutting out the medications from behind with my pen first, so I didn't have to use my fingers and wrists as much. Though my right hand remained numb around the 3rd and 4th fingers, joints and vulnerable; I soon, at least, adapted and got some control over the hand situation, and began to avoid the more serious inflammation and pain. I could pass medications once again and do the g-tube feedings without much trouble.

However, then things got worse. I noticed I felt much more tired than usual, extremely exhausted, and my feet and groin areas became the next target areas of attack. The intermediate unit I worked on required a lot of walking up and down the hallways and in and out of rooms. The soles of my feet and toes became very red, painful and swollen, then numb and barely movable at one point. Often due to pain or a "kink" of sorts in the groin areas, I had to walk with a limp, one day limping on the left, the next day or so, limping on the right. Warm baths and rest helped some, but fatigue had somehow consumed me. And, I just couldn't stop worrying about my feet. I knew that they could use a good, long vacation.

My dear father, a late in life diagnosed diabetic, left behind a glucometer when he passed away, so I did occasionally check my blood for high blood sugar, a sign of diabetes. But I was usually between 70 and 90, which is pretty good. So I didn't worry about this as a problem. While agonizing about my feet, and trying to walk without a limp, I also continued to try hard not to stress out my hands too much, to keep them from flaring up.

On one of the earlier medical appointments, the doctor made sure she ruled out rheumatic fever, since I had struggled through a serious bout of strep throat. It's another occupational hazard, working in a nursing home. I usually did okay if I drank lots of Sunny Delight and got my rest. But, I remember feeling run down before I came down with that nasty bug, probably from working overtime! Another occupational hazard. Somebody calls off and that's it. If nobody answers the phone, it's another four to eight hours of work before any needed rest is possible.

With ongoing problems, and an initial possible diagnosis of polymyalgia rheumatica, which includes pain, often sudden, in the shoulder and hip areas, I was supposedly beyond my doctor's scope. I was referred to a rheumatologist. I made the appointment, but specialists, I guess, are so extremely busy, it seemed ridiculous that I'd have to wait for two months to see someone. By the time the appointment came around, I thought what's the point? A lot of damage could have occurred during that long wait. I was told later, the idea is to simply coordinate management of care with two doctors, a family physician and a rheumatologist.

Due to my health obstacles, I made some changes, took advantage of a job opening closer to home, the night shift, a job with a lower census, so I could sit down and rest more often, and most importantly, a light medication pass so I did not have to stress out my fingers and hands. That was the good news. The bad? It meant I'd lose my insurance, and I couldn't hang onto the previous because the monthly rate was so expensive. Even the two or three days of work a week were very difficult to manage.

My primary doctor had taken some blood tests, but about the only thing that showed up was an elevated sedimentation rate, which supposedly denotes inflammation. Apparently, the ESR, erythrocyte sedimentation rate, is an indirect measure of inflammation. A lab test measures the distance, in millimeters, that red blood cells "settle" in a tube of blood in one hour. If reactants are within the blood, such as asymmetrical proteins, fibrinogens, and gamma globulins, this causes cells to settle more rapidly. (14)

One weekend, someone quit at work, and I needed more money for bills. I offered to work three days in a row. I called my doctor and explained that a flare-up could probably be avoided if I had some prednisone as a preventive protective action plan. But she refused, said I was getting too dependent on it. I said, "Well, I'd better have something, because my feet are killing me again and I know my hands will act up."

She recommended a strong anti-inflammatory medication. I agreed to try it. Huge mistake, a very harmful one. So many meds warn a person not to take it if allergic to aspirin. Well, I'm allergic to aspirin. It makes me wheeze. But I had taken another product, ibuprofen, and managed okay. It got rid of headaches quickly, and I only wheezed slightly only if I took more than two at a time, which I rarely had to do. So when this new med was suggested, I figured, if it didn't agree, my body would let me know, a little wheezing and I'd stop. (By the way, I can no longer take ibuprofen. Now, even one pill makes me wheeze.)

With the first dose, it seemed like magic, the foot pain had subsided. I felt so lucky, figured a medication besides prednisone could help me. After the fourth dose, however, an adverse reaction occurred. Standing at work by the med cart, I felt funny all of a sudden. My left leg and right arm began to go numb. Some red blotches erupted. Just my whole body, I knew something was wrong. I quickly went over to my backpack, got out the antihistamines and took three of them. I told Kelly, the nursing assistant on duty, that I did not feel well. That I thought I'd be fine. "But if anything happens, don't panic, call the ER (emergency room) of the hospital," which was located directly across the street, "and call Micky" the assistant director of nursing, who lived nearby. She seemed to understand what to do if necessary and took all of the information in stride.

That evening, at work, I turned 49. Nurses, especially single ones, we're always working holidays. My life changed on that fateful birthday, with that adverse reaction to a medication. I got through work. I went home and cried and crashed. I knew my life and my health would probably never be the same. I thought about all those years, surviving allergy and asthma attacks, and no serious damage, how lucky I was to have reversible airways, an immune system that would return to normal at times so I could at least have more healthy days. And how on that night, my luck had perhaps changed.

For an allergic/asthmatic, you have to understand, that we don't play sick. And we don't like to miss out on things. Sickness has interfered with so many things already. The missed school days, field trips, parties or special events, lost days of work, the lost days in general because of the sick days. The next day, on Sunday, I had somewhere I needed and wanted to be, so that's just where I headed.

Still not feeling well, still that fuzzy-headed, warm feeling and a right arm irritating me to death with its tingling, swelling, and sensitivity; I thought about telling one of my friends at the meeting that I didn't feel well, just in case, here's my brother's number. And, by the way, I'm allergic to aspirin AND this other medication, and I'm an asthmatic. (I need to get that Medic Alert updated, don't I?) But I thought, what kind of a worry is that to saddle someone with? I just wanted to carry on and enjoy the meeting and be there like I had promised and was supposed to be.

I had continued to take the antihistamines, one every four hours, so I was hoping my arm would clear up at any time. Instead, more bizarre problems occurred on my drive home. The drive should have taken me one hour. With music playing as usual, darkness set in as I traveled north toward home. I just kept driving along and when I decided to look down at the clock in my car, the time on it scared me to death. "That can't be right," I said out loud to myself. "That just can't be right. Something's wrong." I began to cry. I looked around and nothing seemed right.

Finally I saw a billboard sign, and I knew. The time was exactly right and I had just driven a half hour down the road without any memory of doing so. I didn't even remember seeing the lights from the entire town, where I usually turn left. Once in a while, sure, I had passed my turn off, but the next thing I saw, mainly a church with a brightly lit up sign, it reminded me that it was time to turn. I didn't remember seeing the church. I didn't remember driving that period of time. Not until I looked down at the clock. I figured, "great," now I won't even be able to drive. (Luckily no future, loss of time episodes occurred.) At the time though, I wondered, what's next?

I found out at work. After I was introduced to a nursing assistant one evening, I kept trying to remember her name. It was a simple name. I'd ask what it was, say it a couple of times, tell myself to remember it, two minutes later, I simply could not remember her name. I asked about four times. The next time I couldn't remember I said I just wanted to know how to spell it. She looked at me like, "Are you kidding me?" Like I said, it was a simple name, a name kind of like Vickie. In nursing, and on the Alzheimer's unit, we call that a short term memory problem. For example, on the Alzheimer's unit, it doesn't matter how many times you tell a resident what day it is, or what your name is, or what time supper is, or how late you work. Five seconds later, you'll be asked the same questions.

A few days later, as my arm continued to drive me nuts, I typed a letter to my doctor. As someone sat next to me at the computer in the library, I asked, "Could I borrow your right arm for just a little while?" While trying to keep my sense of humor, I actually worried how I would be able to carry on with an arm that felt so weird. After I left there, with tears rolling down my cheeks, I stormed over to the doctor's office to deliver it, the message, that I'D LIKE MY ARM BACK NOW! AND THAT'S MY TENNIS ARM, BY THE WAY!

It wasn't a matter of blame, just very sad circumstances which would probably affect me for the rest of my life. I knew prednisone was only a temporary solution. But I also realized it would have prevented reoccurring symptoms that night at work and that the corticosteroid medication I had asked for, which is the drug of choice often for something like this, would NOT have caused this tragedy. Yet, I am also fully aware of the problems related to the ongoing use of corticosteroids and the very real dangers the doctor tried to stress and avoid on my behalf.

With no health insurance, and wishing I could see that rheumatologist or at least an allergist, I wondered again, just how I would manage. Car troubles of course, never stopped, so as I worked and tried to pay bills, and pay for car repairs as needed, there really wasn't any money for doctors, certainly not specialists who are expensive and usually require many initial diagnostic tests. That was the other reason I didn't rush off to a rheumatologist. Mostly at the initial time because I knew I was about to lose my insurance, since I knew I could not continue to work the one job in Monticello. I didn't have a dependable car to drive the distance and I wasn't healthy enough to drive there anyway.

Also, I read how often thousands and thousands of dollars are spent and nothing shows up. I've been an allergic with a hypersensitive immune system my entire life. In all honesty, it doesn't even take one test to remind me that there are wild and crazy antibodies running around in my body. (Sorry Henry.) I could prove that with the first missed antihistamine dose and touch of a speck of dust or a playtime with my dogs. Let me try and get through three days of heavy med passes without anti-inflammatories, and a picture *will* be worth a thousand words. (For clarification here, I have to apologize to Henry, my imaginary friend, for calling him wild and crazy. Henry is a helpful little antibody who has saved my life many times.)

I can do a real live experiment for anyone that doubts this stuff. Just a quick reminder about another often misunderstood or underestimated etiology, allergies are the 6th leading cause of chronic disease in the U.S. and costs the health care system 18 billion dollars annually. (15) The cost to the individual affected is beyond words.

So anytime. If someone wants to use my body for an experiment, no problem. Rather than after I'm dead and gone, I donate my live, hypersensitive body to science right now. Just don't expect me to stay off the antihistamines and anti-inflammatories for very long, because I'll end up in big trouble real fast. I don't like being dependent on drugs. Like a diabetic, though, I do accept it. If I can live a relatively normal life by correcting my out of balance hyper-immune system with a couple boxes of meds from the dollar store, then I'd be extremely foolish not to do just that.

Oh I forgot to tell you. I got lucky again after that bad luck. A neat nursing assistant at work, Candy, one night after the drug allergy incident, she clued me in about an anti-inflammatory that had helped her. I was scared to death to try anything else, but my feet and toes were still killing me. Again, just like magic, with the very first dose, the pain subsided. I knew they'd be back to normal in no time. Naturally, I feared the second, and third, and especially fourth dose of the new medication; but after a few days, I breathed easy, and I sure walked a lot easier too. Thank God. And Candy. Though caution again, is necessary with the use of medications. Anti-inflammatories can produce adverse side effects, so there are risks with this plan of action.

Winter finally ended and warmer weather shined through. Company arrived, as my stepdaughter, Kassy, her husband, and her two kids came to stay for a while during the summer of 2001. Little Addie sure kept us all busy, running around chasing her or trying to keep her busy until a nap or bedtime. Hard times continued though, due to the fact that I just couldn't work much and yet my car sure didn't understand that I didn't have money to spend on it. Eventually I absolutely had to buy a different car. Kassy and I had fun reconnecting for a couple of months.

Unfortunately though, my health again took a turn for the worse, with a new problem. Realizing the physical stress aspect of the problem, I told Kassy and Addie, that I was sorry, but I wouldn't be able to pick Addie up anymore. Picking her up, holding her on my left side, and taking out a lot of extra bags of trash seemed to be a precursor to a pain that developed in my upper, outer left chest area. It kept getting worse. I was scared. Every day, to wake up, and there it was, PAIN. And it was the kind of pain that you know something is very wrong. And it would get worse with any, any kind of physical and or mental stress. Kassy and her husband were not getting along, and financially, I couldn't help anyone at the time, so I let her know she would have to figure out something else. I felt badly then, and I still do, that I couldn't do more to help. And again, there I was, looking healthy. So how can anyone understand what it's like to live with something as awful, as debilitating as this?

By late July, I tried to hope and pray that it was still only temporary, not permanent damage. It's hard to put something like this into words. All I can say is, I don't know how I made it through those days. I really don't. If you imagine bad, it was much worse. At one point, I even had to turn off the music. I think, and dream, and plan, etc. when I hear music. It makes me feel like dancing. Music inspires me. I couldn't handle *any* stress, bad or good, bad news, bad luck, inspirational excitement, or otherwise. Things had to be canceled. More disappointments. When the end of July arrived, all I could do is work the few days I could, rest, wake up, try and make it through the day, and rest some more. I couldn't do much of anything.

I remember my doctor, early on, stating I could go on disability.

I said, "Disability? You think I can live like this? I can't live like this. I can't do anything. I can't even *think* about doing anything, or the pain in my chest area gets worse. No. I'm going to get better. I have to."

Somehow I knew, for me anyway, I had to keep moving. Believe me, one thing I surely could not have handled, was someone from the welfare office, telling me I didn't look a bit sick, especially when they did a little investigating and found out I still played tennis, walked dogs everyday, and liked to ride a bike! Again, I may look like the healthiest person in the world, but it doesn't mean that my body parts are working right or without pain and limitations.

And even if I did try that, it meant giving up my job because even part-time and I probably made too much money. And to be honest, it was at work, when I had my mind on the job, that I could get my mind off of the pain for a while. No, I decided to keep right on going with my life, and my dreams. Although, of course it had to be at a much slower pace.

My sister and nephew ended up in a crisis situation themselves when they were asked to move because that rental property was being sold. It was a real tough time for my sister and she had always been there for me, so I decided sick or not, I was going to be there for her. I couldn't go to the writers' workshop anyway, as sick as I was. I had a station wagon and it came in handy. I didn't lift anything and made sure I took it real easy. We got her all moved out. Then I went home that day.

I went to bed to rest. I rested and rested. Pain meds never did get rid of it or I probably would have called for a prescription. It didn't matter. I was too sick to drive to go pick it up. My family, they all had their own things going on. The hospital? I could not have handled the stress and they couldn't *see* how critically sick I felt, anyway. At home it was peaceful. I had my sweet dogs nearby. I could be at peace. I could rest, and rest. And hope and pray that the pain was temporary, not permanent, and localized, not causing chaos or permanent damage throughout my whole body.

I imagined healthier times. I fought like I always did when sickness took over. And I waited. If it had gotten any worse, I would have called the ambulance, gone where I needed to be. But for me, it was a personal decision, to try first at home. Sickness, ongoing chronic pain, financial difficulties and car troubles on top of everything; it wears a person down. Trying to work toward and hang onto dreams and the reality of healthier times while feeling sicker than ever before. Hope there's a tomorrow that's just a little easier than today. In reality, there's nothing else to do at the time, but to let it all go for a while, and wait, which I did many times, especially those last few days in July, the summer of 2001.

Enter, Lance Armstrong, his picture on my wall. In my weaker moments, you kept me going Lance Armstrong. Why? We have something in common, reversible symptoms. We're among the lucky ones and we know it. That's why every day's always an extra special day for "us," meaning you, me, all other fighters and survivors of diseases which try to win us over, but so often fail because we put up the strongest fight possible. And since that photo of yours and that dream of mine kept me going, I'll be repaying that favor, in September, when I keep the dream alive. My T-shirt, as I bicycle coast to coast will say, "LEAD THE WAY, LANCE! We're right behind you!   Hypersensitive and autoimmune disease survivors!"

I postponed the trip once already. Couldn't get rid of the pain. I'm better now though, not all better, but getting stronger every day. I've gotten rid of the thoracic pain twice, once in February, once in April, for a whole week at a time. And now, when it does come off and on, it's easier to get rid of. I've let go of the fear of it. It's fear that could have done a lot of damage too, disabled me and my dreams. That was the first thing I tried to let go of when I got sick! Otherwise, afraid to move a sore muscle, it would have frozen me up, immobilized my whole body a long time ago. A friend from church, she's got arthritis. I asked her for her best advice. Elaine said just to "keep moving." So that's exactly what I did, exactly what I still do.

Winter zoomed by and springtime's here again, at last. This hot, sunny summer of 2003, I'll be swimming over at Culver beach. You see I'm still typing. Not without problems since I now do work full-time as a nurse again. But I'm managing. The director of nursing where I work has helped by understanding that I can't work the unit with the heavy med pass more than three days in a row. The Alzheimer's unit saved me, by the way. If not for that, I would have been forced to cut down to part time as more episodes of rheumatoid arthritis and/or carpal tunnel syndrome swollen hands, fingers, and wrists flared. Keep subjecting vulnerable parts of a body to repetitive physical stress, and they are going to suffer. At some point, permanent damage can and will occur. That's certainly a great concern, the possibility of disability or that a particular job must go. Then what?

Doctors? Well, the rheumatologist route, I tried. I was so excited, finally an appointment. I gathered up a chronological list of problems, my history with this stuff and that March 16, 2001 drug reaction episode, everything. Even signed over one of my books, *Sneezing Seasons*, to my new "Partner in Health." Of course I signed it "Henry," that friendly antibody who likes to tell the inside story.

However, fate intervened again. A time change just days before the appointment meant I was late. I explained how I had driven two hours and I really didn't know the time change had gone in effect. I thought maybe the doctor could spare five minutes. But he couldn't. Relayed the message via the nurse that there wasn't really anything he could do for me in five minutes. I thought, well, you could have given me five minutes. So I told the nurse to tell the good doctor that I'd just take care of myself. What good is it going to do me anyway, if I need a doctor, and I can't see him or her for two or three months? I wanted a family doctor, someone who can get to know me, all of my health issues, just an old-fashioned doctor to be there when I needed him or her.

I'm really lucky too, that I didn't waste my time and go back, because that would have been my only visit with him. That doctor got married and moved to Ohio. It made me realize again how important it is to have a family doctor, someone who does have time to get to know the patient and hopefully will be there, at least for years to come.

I did run into another doctor along the way that I liked and he pointed out another important stress factor to consider and work on to lessen the total stress load upon my body and mind. It's called the Thoracic Outlet Syndrome, deals with poor posture, and the wear and tear and age causes of disease and distress such as osteoarthritis and osteoporosis and nerves being compressed, which could account for problems radiating down the arm, via the nerves, perhaps even the dull, but problematic chest pain that sent me to the hospital one night. Pain still occurs at times, after a few consecutive days of work, especially with my left forearm. The median nerve is now giving me problems as well as the ulner nerve at the elbow site.

In the last few weeks, while working the three days in a row with the heavy med pass, I have doubled up on my medication to see if I can avoid further problems. If not, I suppose it will be time to find some type of work in which I do not have to use my hands as much.

Or better yet, let me sell my books! That's on my agenda too. Did you know only six percent of writers make a living at it? (Just in case you think it's strange that I still work a more normal like job.)

All I know is, I do have to save my hands for the daily rituals of dressing, eating, etc., as well as for writing (typing) books. I have used a tape recorder in the past on some projects. However, when I write, I need to be able to change things around, see it in print, things like that. It just doesn't ramble off with a first draft. I write better with my fingers, than with my voice. To backtrack, at least I got something positive from Doctor Purdy, regarding the thoracic pain possibility and posture problems and some greatly needed help one time when my left shoulder suddenly flared up.

I had to run to the hospital previously for excruciating shoulder pain, and once for chest pains. I wanted to avoid that, if I could. Most emergency staff is nice and helpful, but a couple of the doctors, I get either a frown, or a patronizing smile when nothing shows up on the X-ray. One evening at work, I was just walking down the hallway and when I started to move my left arm I realized I couldn't lift it. I just screamed out because any kind of movement and it was unbearable, I mean unbearable pain right at the shoulder joint and down the arm around the deltoid muscle.

Again, I had something to do the next day, and I wasn't going to miss it. But I sure did wonder how I would attend. I didn't want to wake up the doctor, so I took two extra-strength tylenol and an antihistamine and went to bed. At five o'clock he answered his beeper, called me right back and helped me out with calling in a prednisone prescription, just to get it under control again.

I made it through some of the morning program, then I offered apologies and told my friend I had to go. My whole body was aching. In the last week, both my elbows had acted up, both my knees, and now the left shoulder. I was hoping I wouldn't get lost on the way home because I sure felt awfully sluggish and foggy-headed, just like that time before. I made it to the pharmacy. I took 60 mg. of prednisone, and followed through with the rest in the following days. Just like always, (although usually it's a little faster), in two days, I felt the healthiest, all over, that I had felt since the last time I had taken prednisone. I just wish I could stay "cured."

(Late Entry: Following that last attack on my left shoulder, everything was okay for a week or so. Then, not so lucky. My left forearm, elbow and hand seem affected, more vulnerable to pain and less tolerant of activity. Yet the grips are of equal strength. Maybe it's temporary, hmm? Funny, I never thought my right arm would be the strong one. Guess I'm real lucky I saved it.)

After that serious shoulder attack episode, that doctor didn't think he was the right one for me though, so he kind of directed me toward the next two doctors I have now, a bone and joint specialist who is more accessible than a rheumatologist, yet educated regarding rheumatoid arthritis, and only twenty minutes away, and lucky me, a family doctor who just happens to be a holistic practitioner, in the best, truest sense of what that word means to me. Dr. Patchburg is a dream come true! So, we're doing those tests finally, to see if the lupus fits, fibromyalgia, or RA, or a combination of RA and osteoarthritis, or TOS, or none of the above, or some, or all of the above.

Guess I'll have to apologize for my implications if it's not lupus (SLE) specifically that I 'm diagnosed with, but I sure do identify with many of the problems associated with an autoimmune disease. Also, I certainly manage my disease just like someone with lupus or rheumatoid arthritis would.

We're all in this together, unfortunately. Maybe the correct diagnosis for me will simply be my old standby, hypersensitivity. I know one thing, if the attacks stay clear of my vital organs, it just means I'm one of the lucky ones, once again.

We hope to also discover the etiology of the inflammation, if not specifically an autoimmune abnormalty. If no autoantibodies, just the hypersensitive connection, there is another reason my body is over-reacting. One theory is an infectious agent, that strep throat precipitating factor and or other bacterial causative agents. Or, maybe it's simply a matter of interacting factors, genetics, infectious agents, environment and/or hormonal effects causing reactions. (16) Of course, it could be both, autoimmunity and hypersensitivity.

An important health education issue to note regarding increased understanding about autoimmunity, is the fact that many people endure strep throat or bacterial infections. Just like many people come in contact with dust or pollen. Yet, it is the hyperactive immune system or autoimmune reactions that causes illness in certain individuals, while sparing others. Without this distorted, over-reactive immune system, I'd be healthy right now!

Apoptosis is another theory and I'm not really sure if I should root for or fear this one. Feel free to look it up on the internet at your local library. Apoptosis deals with programmed cell death. Over the years, "scientists have found that just as cells weigh many signals in deciding when to grow and divide, they similarly struggle with their very will to live. Each cell, in effect, carries a dagger with which to kill itself when told it is irretrievably damaged or no longer needed." (17)

In other words, for the greater good, to spare someone further disease, cells sacrifice themselves, so disease does not spread. Yet sometimes the process overdoes it, then you wind up with excessive cell death. The field of immunology is absolutely fascinating! Someday, many diseases, right along with autoimmunity and cancer, will no longer exist because researchers will determine how to "re-program" our immune system activity. Seems to be happening right now!

I did get a little confused though when I read the one article, "Death by Design," from the University of Chicago Magazine. Much literature supports the inflammatory process with relation to Alzheimer's and other diseases. This article mentioned neurodegenerative disorders like Alzheimer's, Parkinsons, Huntingtons's, and Lou Gehrig's disease and stated that: "These afflictions draw apoptosis researchers because programmed cell death is so obviously involved, and in each case, nerve cells succumb with a suspicious *lack of inflammation*." (18)

And cancer, I thought maybe this was the answer for cancer too, counterattack any inflammation early on, maybe it would help. Maybe it *would* help some. But listen to this from the book *The Body is the Hero*. Years ago, a "tragic mistake" was made. During a transplant operation, a cancerous kidney was transplanted into a healthy subject. The subject, was of course, on immunosuppressive drugs, in case his immune system decided to reject the new kidney. Well, the patient, in a matter of days, developed a cancerous tumor, then a day later another mass on the other lung. Needless to say, he went back to the operating room. The cancerous kidney was discovered, and the metastatic cancer that had apparently spread from the cancer in the kidney.

Immunosuppressive therapy came to a halt. As the immune system began to function adequately again, the cancer began to disappear. Sadly, along with rejecting the cancer, the transplanted kidney began to get rejected too. The patient had to remain off of immunosuppressive meds. The cancer disappeared, the kidney operation failed, and the patient had to go back on dialysis. (19) What this implies is that the immunosuppressed would be at a higher risk for cancer. A hypersensitive immune system and/or properly working one, it seems to be the better defense against cancer. Fascinating story, isn't it?

Back to *my* symptoms and with regard to my sickness, I do know this much. A red-looking butterfly floated across my face many times within the last year and a half. (This is a classic sign of lupus.) I think it's a heat regulation problem. I've always gotten flushed easily. When I was a little girl practicing acrobatics, I always got severe headaches and Santa Claus-suit red in the face upon exertion and exercise-induced asthma, another chronic disease caused by a hypersensitive immune system. Of course, I endured allergic asthma too, since I've always ranked high on the allergy-prone list. Funny how exercise or physical activity seems to be an antigen with those of us who have these wild and crazy immune systems that like to overreact when it is not necessary.

Also, the arthritis (or arthritis-like) new symptoms began at a time in my life when hormonal changes were taking place which may have contributed to depleted hormonal resources of some immunosuppressive kind necessary to continue to suppress my already hyper-immune system.

I read that a strep throat infection often precedes symptoms like the ones I incurred. I had a painful strep throat infection. I saw the white spots in my throat. There was an outbreak of strep at the nursing home at the time. Shortly after, my hands, the same hands and fingers I had always used to pass medications, just couldn't do it anymore. Not without swelling up twice the size that they should have been, not without the excruciating pain. The groin area kinks, the problem with my toes and feet, and acute attacks of pain in the shoulders also, even abdominal pains at times, the sudden loss of hair at the baseline; these all occurred about four weeks after the strep infection.

The upper, outer left thoracic chest pain, it came later. It occurred after lifting, using those pectoral muscles. To this day, any type of physical stress causes problems, either in my hands, shoulders, feet, or manifests afterwards as a systemic extremely fatigued feeling. Even the thoracic pain. It's gone, I'm free of it. Then, the next thing I know, after some physical stress, carrying something or mental stress, when I begin to try and write a chapter in a book, a lot is going on in my head, here it comes. It's back. I think "Oh, Oh." But then I just go about my business. Later on, I'll notice, it's gone. Or the next morning when I wake up, I get lucky and I think, all right, a thoracic pain free day.

As far as differences to osteoarthritis and the rheumatoid caused type? It's no surprise that women approaching fifty years old, might develop signs and symptoms of osteoarthritis, even osteoporosis, especially if corticosteroids have played a role in the history of a person. It's also not surprising that someone ill seeking help, may have a number of health problems coexisting. I learned, however, that there are distinguishing features between the two types of arthritis, osteo and rheumatoid. Rheumatoid tends to be symmetrical, occurring on equal sides of the body, such as right elbow, left elbow, right knee, left knee. Also, the knuckle areas closest to the fingertips are usually not affected. (20) That occurs in osteoarthritis, the wear and tear kind. I see it all the time in the elderly population. The knuckles closest to my fingertips were not affected. Acute flare-ups occurred and then went into remission. I developed symmetrical problems, whenever one side of my body acted up, the other side followed.

Here's another fact. Immunosuppressive drugs suppress my over-reactive immune system and I feel well again. Anti-inflammatory medications, also, they counteract some process that is taking place as I try to work and/or do other things with my hands and feet and body and mind. In my opinion, as well as many others I've read about, anecdotal facts are certainly worth paying attention to.

My eyesight seems to be worsening. When I've used my hands quite a bit in a day, either typing or at work, the veins in my hands sure do become a lot more visible and seem to be popping out of my skin. I read where veins are not usually affected, but mine sure do seem to flare up. I wonder about the effects of inflammation upon blood vessels which affect the eyes, brain, heart, whole body. I also often wonder about how many strokes and knowledge and memory deficiency problems might be prevented by early counteraction of inflammation.

I ask you, what is happening to me? Mysterious malady, or an autoimmune related disease process, or a combination of disease processes? I know I have a hyper-sensitive immune system. Whatever name or label is given to the cause of the symptoms, I know it relates partly to the fact that I have those wild and crazy rebel antibodies running around inside causing havoc at times. (I just hope Henry and I can just stay one step ahead of them and keep on counterattacking.)

Just one more reminder, one more fact. My first symptoms began with *physical* stress upon body parts, *physical* stress. A carpal tunnel syndrome-like attack can be one of the first symptoms of an autoimmune disease. (21) To this day, any and every healthcare practitioner in the world could offer suggestions for me to change things. I might improve my nutrition, trump up my daily exercise, practice more stress management tips, resolve any conflicts; but if my immune system is NOT suppressed, as I use my fingers, hands, wrists, legs, feet, etc., there will be adverse effects. Free me of every mental stressor in my life. Give me one physical stress factor, and I WILL have to pay the consequences, unless I manage, by suppression, the real culprit, this out of control hypersensitive immune system causing the havoc.

When I asked for help, a doctor once said to me regarding the hypersensitive and hormonal connection theories, *"If you believe that, then I might not be able to help you."* He acted like he really wanted to help too. I didn't say anything at the time. I thought, doesn't he realize that some people are born like this? We deal with hypersensitivity our whole lives? Then when we mention it as a plausible, logical assumption, to think that it might just all be related somehow, we get looked at like we're crazy? But if the doctor didn't believe in these causative factors, even if only some of it was related to my hormonal changes and hypersensitivity, then there was no "might" about it. He couldn't help. It worries me that we still have a long, long way to go regarding understanding, preventing and properly treating timely, serious hormonal imbalances, allergies, asthma, hypersensitivity and autoimmune diseases, which are all immune system related.

Although with allergic reactions, it will be important to remember that there must be a true antigen-antibody reaction. With autoimmunity, if the essential key element is not there, self-attacks, we should not label the reactions as autoimmune. Otherwise, like so many other disorders, before you know it, everyone's walking around saying, I have this mysterious disorder, it's called autoimmune disease. Just like MS in kids, we don't want to miss a diagnosis, but we don't want to use a handy diagnosis excessively either, unless there is just cause. I believe for the most part, initially, I stated that I had many of the symptoms of lupus. One time, however, due to a busy day, and simplification of the matter, I did respond to a co-worker by saying, "Systemic," when she asked me what kind of lupus I had.

Maybe I should have just stuck with the diagnosis and words, "a wild and crazy, over-reactive immune system." When people ask me, "What's wrong with your wrists?" It just seems easier to say arthritis, than to explain possible autoimmune reactions and the fact that if I don't take meds and wear the supports or if I overdue it, my wrists, fingers, and joints go haywire and then I can't use them at all until I dose myself up with prednisone to tone down the agonizing, debilitating symptoms.

My heart goes out to anyone struggling with any of these debilitating signs and symptoms. Please remember that permanent damage may be prevented if you act quickly. You may have to make changes, occupational or otherwise, in your life. Mostly, you will have to decide what really helps and what does not. Good health and time are two of the most precious things on earth. Enjoy, and the best of luck.

One last mention of something very important. There was another doctor who I came across that didn't seem to believe I had a serious problem at all, even after I explained all of my symptoms and all of the disabled days I was encountering. I left him a pamphlet regarding autoimmune diseases too. He didn't seem to even believe me when I told him about my adverse reaction to that med I took. Again, I kind of wished for a clubbed foot, or missing limb or something visibly wrong with me. I thought about letting my hands flare up so he could see them in their swollen, diseased state. But I decided against that, just to move on because like I told the doctor, "I don't stay where I'm not welcome."

But what occurred in that medical office between that doctor and myself, I know that it probably happens far too often. I explained how ill I had been and asked for basic tests to see if my thyroid was working right, if my sedimentation rate was normal or high, a urinalysis, to make certain my kidneys were okay. I said, just think of it as a wellness check. He said he didn't like to do a lot of unnecessary tests, unless there seemed to be a real need or indication for them. Well, usually I agreed. No need to take advantage of the elderly or sick or disabled like some unethical medical people do, more diagnostic tests, more visits, more costs.

However, this *was* an instance to act, to diagnose, to help. Whenever I brought up the autoimmunity issue, the doctor cringed. It was like philosophical medical irreconcilable differences between us. I realize it's baffling, not to see much inflammation, to simply go by what is reported. But I have to wonder if a surgeon or pilot, tall and male, had walked in and explained the same exact symptoms and the fact that they couldn't do their jobs, perform important surgeries or fly an airplane full of passengers safely with swollen up disabled hands; would they have been taken more seriously perhaps? There seemed to be some other quick solution that fit to describe my age-related problems. I kept explaining, or trying to, that it wasn't merely aches and pains and expecting to feel like a "spring chicken" anymore. *"When the flare-ups happen, these are disabling symptoms, disabling. And that upper, outer chest pain Doctor, I don't know how I lived with it."*

I told him, he couldn't see how difficult my life had been due to these rheumatoid-arthritis like attacks, but it has caused some permanent damage and I wanted to prevent any more. Also, I don't think he realized how lucky I was to still be able to work. For a while I barely got through part-time work days, and that's all I could do. It has been an incredibly tough challenge to continue working with these serious health problems. The doctor didn't seem to understand any of what I told him or pay attention to the long list of serious symptoms I had described.

I have a friend also, Amber, and she told me how her doctor just kept looking at her like she was crazy. This one I don't understand because Amber's mother has suffered with lupus for years, and her sister. The predisposition runs in families. And yet, still, her problems were shrugged off as a female with some kind of inner psychological problems that if only faced, her fingers and hands and wrists would magically start working properly again. Well, both Amber and I are very grateful, because we know how very lucky we are to be able to still use our hands. We really do. Some victims who were ignored, in their earlier stages of over-reactive immune system diseases were not so lucky.

So instead of the diagnostic tests I asked for to see what was happening internally, with this one doctor, he repeated a question several times. *"What's your worst fear, but, what's your worst fear?"* And I'm thinking, didn't I explain that already? The fact that some minor permanent damage has occurred already, and more might have occurred or might to my vital organs, if I can't stop this disease process.

Again, *"But what's your worst fear?"* Well, since I left that doctor and moved on long ago, I've had a lot of time to think about that question. So I'll answer it here.

My biggest/worst fear(s) probably relate to the following: the fear that illness or an accident could hurt someone I love or care about, future wars or terrorism could hurt us, natural disasters could strike, like tornadoes, etc. And this.

I am terrified that someone suffering from all of the extremely serious and disabling symptoms such as mine will walk into a doctor's office and *not* be taken seriously. The doctor will not act quickly enough. That patient, whether a two or ten year old, a teenager, or an adult woman, or even man, will then have to find more doctors to try and get to the root of their problems. Years will pass, and all the while, due to hypersensitive or autoimmune reactions allowed to continue out of control, permanent damage will occur. Quality of life will be lost, and in some cases, just like Ricky, or Amy, Angela, Anne, my cousin, or thousands of others, because a disease process was able to win the race against time and ineffective life-saving healthcare, needless, painful disability will occur, or more people will die. Does that answer your question doctor?

Days, hours are important to us. Years of neglect and misunderstanding we cannot afford. If we allow that, then we may end up dead, as many victims are, certainly disheartened and/or disabled like many more victims.

Again, "We may be sick at times, but we are not weak." I might add, we are fighting for our lives, so rest assured, we are fighting against our signs and symptoms as hard as we can. But we cannot do it without a lot of help. Sometimes we also make mistakes or let valuable time pass before following an effective healthcare action plan. But, as long as we do our part too, medical professionals have the potential to prevent disability and death, and give us the support we need. I hope we can all grow stronger, healthier, and wiser together.

I should mention that the doctor I just spoke about sent me an apology in writing, which I gladly accepted. He realized some limitations in dealing with patients and wished me luck. I wrote back and told him thanks, and confessed, that yes, sometimes I can be a "little" difficult to deal with as a patient, especially at first. But I try hard to be healthy and just need a partner in health, a doctor to understand my hypersensitive body, hang in there with me, so I can prevent further damage and stay as healthy as possible.

CHAPTER TWO

Who This Book is For

This book is for all sufferers and survivors of autoimmune diseases or for anyone experiencing the debilitating attacks of abnormal alarmist antibodies. For you, the late Dr. Norman Cousins, one of my heroes, victim and survivor of ankylosing spondylitis. Your books and your life inspired me. For you, my dear friend, Anne, a true modern day hero. Multiple Sclerosis, your affliction, may have stolen your body, but it certainly never won your heart or mind or incredible ongoing curiosity about life. For your friend Julie too Anne, the lucky one that obtained an early diagnosis and began to halt the autoimmune process.

For you Montel Williams, Annette Funicello, cousin Lorraine; and anyone else with multiple sclerosis, I hope MS never destroys your hearts and souls either. And you, dear nephew Kenneth, victim and fighter of a serious autoimmune disease, and beloved sister who appears afflicted, this book is for you too!

Autoimmunity Counterattack is also for Virginia T. Ladd, another honored acquaintance, victim and survivor of lupus, and founder of The American Autoimmune Related Disease Association. For you Kellie Martin and Leah Ross and your sisters, Heather and Heidi, all of you, for your bravery to counterattack against the adverse affects of autoimmunity.

This book is for all the faces and lives affected, or claimed, by out of control autoimmune diseases. This book pays tribute and remembers you! AMY, who died from hemolytic anemia and autoimmune thrombocytopenia at the age of 16 years old. LEAH, a young fighter battling five autoimmune diseases. For you RICKY, innocent two year old who never seemed to have a chance.

Also, for you, ANGEL, forever gone at the age of 18 from lupus nephritis. Since little progress has been made to prevent or counteract this disease progress in decades; you never seemed to have a chance either.

For you too, Audrey Kron, a courageous soldier and teacher in this war. You fought long and hard. We will always remember you. Condolences to your family and friends. May your written words of wisdom encourage us all, for years to come, to continue our fight toward optimal health.

For other authors who have shared their stories, their journeys into the dark land of sickness and back again to bathe in the healing sunlight, to Montel Williams, Mary J. Shoman, John Merchant (ankylosing spondylitis survivor), and all of the others, thanks for caring and sharing.

My heart goes out to Jenna, Drew, Halley, Kate, and a friend of mine, Amber, and her family, all survivors who suffer from autoimmunity. My sister's friends too, Betsy, and the others.

My heart and this book also wants to acknowledge the arthritically challenged, the kids who suffer juvenile rheumatoid arthritis, and to every sweet middle-aged or elderly lady and gentleman out there in the world who must deal with the painful reality of arthritis. We all have something in common. We suffer from autoimmunity and/or abnormally hypersensitive immune systems. I hope we all can continue to fight with all of our might to combat our diseases and enjoy optimal health.

For the lupus victims and survivors, I hope this book helps to increase understanding about this disease too, partly because I seem to suffer many of the same symptoms of SLE, (eight out of ten yes answers on the test yourself for Lupus scoreboard by the LFA.) When our hair falls out, when excruciating burning pain and tingling sensations or numbness plagues us, when we begin to overheat and our brains act sluggish, when that flushed reddened butterfly floats across our faces and our joints, muscles or organs begin to fail us; let's hope that at the very least, people understand that a very real, threatening disease exists within. Rather than doubting us because we might look or even feel healthy at times; let's ask the healthcare profession to kindly take us very seriously, listen to our signs and symptoms; and quickly help to save our quality of life, in the more serious cases, our lives.

To the Mr. And Mrs. there in Portage, Indiana doing such a fine job for the Lupus Foundation of America on a familiar local basis for the area in which I live, hang in there and keep up the good work. It's so important!

For fibromyalgia and chronic fatigue victims and survivors, you are not forgotten. The way you search for answers too, the way you survive day after day always fighting the symptoms, amid the adversity which you face. I know what your symptoms feel like too, I've endured many of them. All I can say is, fight on. These disease processes are demanding insight, understanding, and improved treatment. Hang onto hope and try your best to keep moving to whatever degree you are able to. Hopefully a turning point will come and life will again be better than you ever imagined possible.

Your diseases may be two of the most difficult and baffling ones for the medical world and family members to comprehend. Help them. There is a great deal of literature which explains the facts and dispels the myths regarding the notion that "it's all in your head." Buy books or search the internet and print up materials, if necessary. Just make sure they are credible ones, not someone trying to sell a bunch of expensive nonsense. Your pain, your fatigue, no matter how you try to counterattack, is real, as you well know. The thing to focus on, is how to rid yourself of it or lessen the severity as much as possible. Unfortunately, the specific causes and answers might be as difficult to "see" as the symptoms experienced at times. If detection of proof is not found, it might help to simply view your problem as a hypersensitive nervous system, with the sensation of pain magnified. Move on to a different level, that of focusing on the disappearance or management of the symptoms. That is the goal.

Too many of these diseases consume our lives. Why? For one thing, that agonizing element of pain takes over. Humans are curious though too. We want to know. We want to understand and make sense of things. Distance ourselves from disease, live in an alternate reality even for a short time, and it could lead to some healthier moments, days, weeks, months, and so on. Disease is not our friend, yet it seems to want our undivided attention all the time. Especially pain, it is often the worst selfish enemy.

For those other millions too, the allergy-afflicted and asthmatics, suffering from hypersensitive immune systems, *Autoimmunity Counterattack* is also written for you! Sneezing and wheezing a person's way through life is awfully difficult too! Just like you, even though you often sit in class, or at work, or at home looking like the healthiest person around; it doesn't negate the facts, the intermittent disturbances and immunological imbalances that come and go. Just like the pain or intermittent signs and symptoms endured by those suffering from autoimmunity, certain health problems may be invisible to others, but it certainly is vividly real to the one suffering. A teacher can't peak into a bedroom window at night and see a student sitting hunched over in bed wheezing and struggling to breathe. A boss may not understand that an employee only got two hours of sleep due to a severe allergy or autoimmune attack the night before. We can't show people a picture of what it was like, unless of course we resort to that nightmare video tape.

Actually, I do believe a picture is worth a thousand words. Maybe it's something to think about. Especially with asthmatic kids or someone dealing with rheumatoid arthritis flair-ups with hands swollen twice the size of normal and handicapped to the point of non-use. Visual effects could work as a terrific health educator.

Hypersensitive individuals, we all have something in common. We want to be healthy. We want to participate and live on without struggling with disabling symptoms which alter our temperaments. We want to live without debilitating or deadly afflictions which may end our dreams too soon.

Chronic pain sufferers/survivors, I truly hope this book eases that overwhelming obstacle in your lives, pain.

Some other particulars. This book is also for you, all the fine, dedicated researchers in the field of allergy and immunology. The family members also, of those who spend long hours trying to help us. Even loved ones in my life, because sometimes the "cause" seems to demand extra hours/effort; and sometimes maybe a heart and mind can't be in two places at one time.

To all healthcare givers, researchers, hospitals, clinics, health educators, associations, funding organizations, politicians, support chapters, parents, teachers, other family and friends willing to stand by and persevere; thank you. We desperately need your support and understanding.

And let's even include the "radicals" too in that important group, because like any researcher, right or wrong; it should be the underlying sincere efforts to discover and help that we should embrace and appreciate. However, when it comes to profit-making money as motivation, or dangerous health fads; conflicts of interest just might exclude some radicals or extremists from deserving the attention they receive. But this book is for all of you, because if quality of life and actual lives are at stake, if you are steering in the wrong direction; perhaps you could change course and come to help us too. We cannot afford wasted time and energy on some bogus "miracle cure" pathway of deception. We need real answers, real cures and proven ways to correct or suppress the malfunctioning or over-reactive immune system attacks which our bodies are encountering.

It is my hope that none of us will suffer in vain, or die or fight, or even live in vain. We should share our stories and know in our hearts that we never stand alone during crisis. Too many millions are experiencing similar, difficult health challenges or setbacks at the same time.

And I can't forget how every remarkable handy capable person I've ever known or heard about has helped to make me stronger. This book is for all of you too.

Especially, I cannot forget the dreamers of the world. Without their inspiration, life would be so dull and routine. The mountain climbers, the sail around the world or fly across the ocean adventurers, the daring hot air balloonists, the creative artistic individuals who never give up, no matter what; and that amazing wonder, Lance Armstrong, and a fellow Hoosier, Jim Stack and his cross-country cycling team, Leah Ross, avid hiker in honor of her sister-all heroes of mine; you all helped me to keep bouncing back and especially encouraged me to keep on dreaming. As far as Lance Armstrong and Jim Stack go, to keep on pedaling. My new inspiring coast to coast cycling partners too! To live amongst persistent dreamers, it is truly an honor.

Of course, crossing the finish line isn't the important thing though. It's being able to dream and participate that means so much to me and anyone who battles a disease or struggles to stay as healthy as possible.

Finally, for all victims and survivors, I hope this book offers you hope, understanding, and strength, to continue to fight with all your might, to adapt, to survive, and to live in the awesome Land of Wellness. Make any limitations you can, disappear. Adapt, cope, and transcend to be as healthy as humanly possible. When you do that, you've conquered fear, pain, and your disease. When you cross those finish lines; you'll enter into another magical zone, called *the realm of possibility*.

CHAPTER THREE

THE HYPERSENSITIVE AND AUTOIMMUNE DISEASE RELATED FACTS OF LIFE

FACT: Autoimmune disease refers to a varied group of more than 80 serious, chronic illnesses that involve almost every human organ system. It includes diseases of all bodily systems as well as the skin and other connective tissues, eyes, blood, and blood vessels. In all of these diseases, the underlying problem is similar-the body's immune system becomes misdirected, attacking the very organs it was designed to protect.

FACT: Although children and men are also affected at times, autoimmune diseases occur in women about 75 % of the time.

FACT: Lupus is a chronic, autoimmune disease which causes inflammation of various parts of the body, especially the skin, joints, blood and kidneys. The immune system normally protects the body against viruses, bacteria and other foreign materials. In an autoimmune disease like lupus, the immune system loses its ability to tell the difference between foreign substances and its own cells and tissues. The immune system then makes antibodies directed against "self."

FACT: Autoimmune and inflammatory diseases cause considerable suffering. Rheumatoid arthritis, multiple sclerosis, type-I diabetes, asthma and inflammatory bowel disease affect more than one-tenth of all people. This figure is even higher if hardening of the arteries and neurodegenerative diseases are included. The progress of all these diseases includes a distinct inflammatory component. What all these diseases have in common is that they more or less selectively attack the function of vital tissues or organs, even completely destroying them sometimes. These diseases feature imbalances in the regulation of inflammatory or immunologically active cells. (22, Activebiotech)

FACT: According to the latest statistics regarding hypersensitive immune systems, from the National Institute of Allergy and Infectious Diseases, estimates suggest that: "Allergies affect as many as 40 to 50 million people in the U.S. Pollen allergy (hay fever) affects nearly 9.3 percent in the U.S., not including those with asthma. Chronic sinusitis, sometimes caused by allergies, affects nearly 35 million people in the U.S. Asthma, a chronic disease of lung inflammation, is on the rise. From 1990 to 1994, the number of people with self-reported asthma in the U.S.

increased from 10.4 million to 14.6 million. Asthma affected an estimated 4.8 million U.S. children in 1994. Currently, asthma is the leading cause of missed school days.

FACT: Understanding and managing the delicate balance of the immune system in order to counteract hypersensitivity or autoimmunity, while still maintaining the body's ability to fight disease, especially while using immunosuppressive medications, is crucial.

FACT: Hormones, genetic components, and environmental risk factors contribute to the causes of these diseases.

FACT: Autoimmune diseases remain among the most poorly understood and poorly recognized of any category of illnesses.

FACT: Lupus, an autoimmune disease, is not contagious, cancerous or related to AIDs, the immunodeficiency disease.

FACT: The Public Health Service Office on Women's Health and other health agencies are providing a solid foundation from which to increase knowledge about autoimmune disorders in women.

FACT: Due to the fact that the diseases affect multiple body systems, symptoms come and go, and are often misleading, which hinders accurate diagnosis.

FACT: Autoimmune diseases range from mild to disabling and potentially life-threatening. Although lupus also ranges from mild to life-threatening, 5,000 Americans die every year, yet the majority of the cases can be controlled with proper treatment. Many lupus deaths can be avoided if the patient is diagnosed early.

FACT: Lupus affects 1 out of every 185 Americans.

FACT: The average lupus patient has symptoms 3 to 10 years prior to diagnosis. Lupus is more prevalent in African Americans, Latinos, Native Americans and Asians.

FACT: Organ specific disorders result when the autoimmune process is misdirected and attacks a person's organs. Tragedies such as permanent damage to organs, joints, tissues, and other parts of the body including the sensory organs such as eyesight, can often be avoided with early diagnosis and adequate medical intervention.

FACT: Non-specific autoimmune disorders are widespread throughout the body, thus labeled systemic.

FACT: Autoimmune diseases occur while women often look healthy.

FACT: Over 45% of patients with autoimmune diseases have been labeled chronic complainers in the earliest stages of their illness.

FACT: Unlike cancer, autoimmunity has not been accepted or labeled as a category of disease.

FACT: According to estimates, autoimmune diseases cost $86 billion dollars per year.

FACT: Correction of all major deficiencies is of utmost importance. Examples would include: replacement of hormones not being produced by glands, insulin in Type I diabetes, replacement of blood by transfusion, and nutritional supplements when warranted by noted deficiencies.

FACT: The American Autoimmune Related Disease Association recognizes the need for more collaboration in research involving autoimmune diseases and the need for more basic research into autoimmunity as the underlying cause of these diseases. This, along with helping to raise physician and public awareness of autoimmunity as a category of disease so that early screening and prevention programs will one day be commonplace, is the primary mission of AARDA.

FACT: While medical science has not yet developed a method for curing lupus, new research brings unexpected findings and increased hope each year.

(22) For references see bibliography

CHAPTER FOUR

The ABC Nursing Care Plan of Action

A. **THE PROBLEM:**

Hypersensitive and autoimmune related signs, symptoms, and complications.

B. **GOAL/OUTCOME**:

To maintain an optimal level of well-being by preventing and counterattacking hyperactive and autoimmune system reactions.

C. **INTERVENTIONS**:

Utilize a holistic approach to education, prevention and treatment. Study and understand the ABCs: Awareness, balance, and commitment.

AWARENESS: Learn about your disease process, acknowledge signs, symptoms, and triggers.

BALANCE: Learn how to regain a healthy balance. Counterattack a hyper/auto-active or dysfunctional immune system. Also, adapt, learn how to regain a healthy balance in your life.

COMMITMENT: Persevere, remain determined, follow through with a health care plan of prevention/counteraction. If setbacks happen, practice resilience and restore a powerful positive attitude of commitment as soon as possible.

NOTE: Outline a care plan for each specific problem.

EXAMPLE:

(A) Problem: Flare-ups in hands, fingers, wrists
(B) Goal/Outcome: Prevent and/or counterattack symptoms
(C) Interventions: Understand triggers, pace self, wrist supports, counteractive meds, exercises, caution as carry/lift

CHAPTER FIVE

The ABC's Toward Wellness:
Awareness, Balance, and
Commitment

A=AWARENESS

To fight any war, a soldier needs to know as much as possible about the enemy. That's common sense, and anyone battling a disease, whether he/she likes it or not, must become a fighter. Understanding the autoimmune disease process, the definition of an autoimmune reaction and the premise of what happens when it occurs, realizing the basics can be easy. It's a matter of how much a person wants to learn which may determine how difficult it is to fully get educated on the subject. For the purposes of this book, I'll try to simplify the topic and accomplish at least a basic understanding of autoimmunity. However, I'll also mention a book and some pamphlets that can be read if more advanced knowledge is desired.

We grow up recognizing the importance of vaccinations to prevent disease. Vaccines work by stimulating our protective immune systems, to make specific antibodies which will attack a particular enemy-disease in the future if the need arises. Bacteria, viruses, microorganisms, those unhealthy germs we fear; we expect our immune systems and antibiotics, whenever necessary, to protect us against foreign invaders. When it works properly, we are grateful for our effective immune defense systems. After all, not everyone is so lucky. Those with immune deficiency diseases cannot protect themselves.

If our immune systems are intact, however, even hypersensitive to the point of over-reacting, at least we can prevent and fight against many diseases. Antibodies are made and come to our rescue. They act as our knights in shining armor, seek out, recognize and destroy the potentially harmful enemy attackers invading our human body. Antibodies counterattack!

With regard to autoimmune diseases, however, something goes haywire. As mentioned in the introduction, antibodies lose the ability to differentiate between truly harmful foreign invaders. Inflammation occurs as war is declared on the self, the body's own cells, tissues, and/or organs. Disabling and/or deadly diseases can follow.

Again, it's a matter of how intricately involved a person wants to get as far as understanding what goes on at this point. But the important thing to understand is that a distorted, harmful process begins due to a dysfuntional immune system. If not suppressed, if no counterattack is set into motion, then the inflammation can continue and permanent damage may result. That's why immunosuppressive and anti-inflammatory drugs work. The out of control, unnecessary over-protective immune system is brought back into balance by suppressing the self-attack within or counteracting the inflammatory process affecting various areas of the body such as: the synovial lining surrounding joints, the nervous system, brain cell area, the tissues, blood vessels, and/or vital organs.

I could elaborate on the immune system cells, explain in more detail about specific duties carried out by the lymphocytes (one type of white blood cell) including T and B cells, true assassinators of infected cells. Or I could delve further into the jobs accomplished by other soldier-like cells, the macrophages and neutrophils patrolling, circulating in the blood and searching for foreign substances.

But the best health educational resources I can think of are already out there. A pamphlet entitled *Understanding Autoimmune Disease* is available free upon request from the National Institute of Health/National Institute of Allergy and Infectious Diseases. Inquire about NIH Publication No. 98-4273, May of 1998, if interested.

Also, if you like story versions instead to illustrate a point, a fictitious friendly antibody named Henry will narrate and tell you the inside story about the immunological wars which take place within allergic, hypersensitive human bodies. A book titled *Sneezing Seasons*, which I wrote years ago might help. It's available at: www.infinitypublishing.com.

Here is a special book too that would probably be very helpful to people with autoimmune diseases. *The Autoimmune Connection* by Rita Baron-Faust and Jill P. Buyon, published by Contemporary Books, McGraw-Hill.

There is one thing to remember though regarding the difference between allergic hypersensitive reactions and autoimmune attacks. Though similar in nature, all due to an unnecessary, out of control immune system, allergic reactions target invading substances, antigens from outside the body. Autoimmune reactions happen when that haywire mechanism kicks in and the immune system can no longer differentiate self from foreign invaders or outside antigens. The misdirected, defective and dangerous immune system then begins to travel down the mistaken pathway of self-destruction.

When this disease process begins, it is critical to understand what is happening and it is imperative to initiate the suppression of hyper-reactive tendencies immediately. If no counterattack is activated, war now declared on a person's very own precious body will continue to damage and destroy healthy anatomical parts. Not only is quality of life threatened, thousands of actual lives are lost every year because an autoimmune victim, for whatever reasons, was not equipped with the necessary "weapons" to counterattack the deadly war within. Once we understand the enemy and the way it works, we can counterattack sooner and more effectively and we will turn this battle around and save lives and/or the quality of life for millions. Of course, ideally, in time, immune deficiencies along with allergic and autoimmune related diseases will (hopefully) be prevented.

Another essential point that I'd like to reiterate is that more accurate line of thinking which views autoimmunity as a cause (etiology) and category of disease. After I gave my brief health educational talk to my 12 year old nephew the other day, I quizzed him afterwards.

I asked, "Now Kris, tell me, if a person has a case of Type I diabetes, what does that person suffer from?"

He gave the usual answer. "Type I diabetes."

"Yes, but what is the main problem, that overall disease process that caused the damage in the pancreas area, so that person cannot lower his or her blood sugar any more? What does the person suffer from? That one simple answer?"

"Oh, autoimmunity." He smiled and I smiled back.

"That's right, you got it. Whether it's attacking the pancreas, thyroid, the vital organs, joints, tissues, or skin, the brain or nervous system; autoimmunity is the problem."

It's time to demystify these immune-related diseases, simplify, educate and better understand what we are dealing with, just what enemy we have to fight against. Terror is often due to the unknown, the secret, merciless attack upon an innocent victim. We cannot fight the enemy, unless we know who or what is attacking us. Just remember though, even the fictitious hero Superman had a weakness. And sometimes beating the enemy simply means discovering who, where, and what the enemy is and facing that same merciless force without fear. Let's look autoimmunity right in the eye and say, "We're not going to take it anymore. This battle we will win. Because as long as we are fighting with all of our might, we already won."

Something else, crucially important to any soldier or survivor of war: utilizing the best, strongest defenses possible. Like a durable fort built to protect, our bodies should be our best defense. In any war there will be factors that cannot be controlled. As victims come under attack, it will be the "forts of steel" that survive. That means that any "ammunition" available should be utilized to the max to strengthen our bodies' defensive capabilities.

How can our bodies become a "fort of steel," impenetrable to dangerous enemies and able to sustain, counterattack, even conquer during battles which confront us? Awareness, balance, commitment.

Included within the awareness armory, lifestyle habits that build strong, resilient bodies and minds. We are already aware of many stress factors that challenge our existence. At this point, I'm going to "stress" one more enemy that we all need to fight against. With increased awareness, I think you'll understand more than ever before how important it is to work on building a strong nutritional defense.

As I attended a lupus support group meeting one evening, the hospital dietician spoke about oxidative stress and free radicals. She even gave us a visual, explained that there is a negative side to oxygen and aging, and disease processes occur because of this enemy. We pictured an apple sliced up and then as exposed to air, turning brown.

That same process, caused by oxidative stress happens to us.

I further researched the culprit and the interesting, but detrimental other enemies called free radicals. According to Dr. Ray Strand, a qualified specialist in nutritional medicine, "The same process that causes a cut apple to turn brown or iron to rust is the cause of all the chronic degenerative diseases we fear and even the aging process itself." After I heard the dietician speak that night and reading about all of this from Dr. Strand, I realized why the health food stores keep talking about free radicals. It dawned on me that it's also the reason doctors are ordering antioxidants (which are thought to reduce the levels of free radical activity) more and more for the elderly. I also learned that "oxidative damage to brain cells may be a valuable indicator of Alzheimer's disease activity. Increased oxidative stress is often associated with tissue inflammation, a long-suspected cause of Alzheimer's disease." (23)

Free radicals. I had heard about these radicals before, but never did fully understand the scope of their adverse effects. Now understood by many as a definite front line enemy to try and avoid or fight against in order to maintain good health; there is a great deal of educating, researching, and counteracting going on to try and help those suffering, as well as urging the prevention of illness by understanding and combating oxidative stress.

Dr. Strand describes a free radical as this: "The free radical has at least one unpaired electron in its outer orbit essentially giving it an electrical charge. If this free radical is NOT readily neutralized by an antioxidant it can go on to create more volatile free radicals, damage the cell wall, vessel wall, proteins, fats, and even the DNA nucleus of our cells." (24) He also paints a picture for us so we can understand the kind of damage that might result. We're asked to think of ourselves sitting in front of a fireplace. Then snap, crackle, pop goes the fire.

"The fire burns safely and beautifully most of the time, but on occasion out pops a hot cinder that lands on your carpet and burns a little hole in it. One cinder by itself doesn't pose much of a threat; but if this sparkling and popping continues month after month, year after year, you will have a pretty 'ratty' carpet in front of your fireplace." (25)

Like the dietician that spoke at the hospital about lupus, free radicals, and powerful combatants called antioxidants; the doctor recommended fruits and vegetables. In a day and age when other enemies to our health are ganging up on us: busy lifestyles, infatuation and reliance of pills, ongoing self-destructive habits such as smoking and drinking, environmental toxins, and social stressors like terrorism; we need to be aware, prevent, and counterattack as much as possible. Better nutrition can be one of our greatest allies. We can strengthen our inner "fort" by creating, ingesting "our own army of antioxidants, which are able to neutralize free radicals and render themselves harmless."(26)

Now I like fast food restaurants as much as the next burger and French fry junkie, but I know I have to prioritize and be more considerate of my health, rather than my cravings. Yet, I've always been a firm believer in moderation. So I don't think we have to cut Burger King and McDonald's out of our diets altogether. But I sure do think we ought to eat there a lot less, add a lot more healthier foods to our diet, and buy their salads more often.

Of course, while we're at it, don't forget that other often neglected vital ally that fights against disease, exercise. Posture too, I missed that support group educational meeting, but I'm sure it's another crucial element that needs increased awareness as a major counteractive measure with regard to inflammatory and immune-mediated neuromuscular and degenerative diseases, which are so painful.

While we're still on the issue of awareness, let me share one more disturbing area of concern, that of environmental toxins. As I researched materials for this book, I stumbled upon what might be one of the most controversial topics of the 21st century. After reviewing both sides of the story, believers and non-believers, I initially began to write and write. But then I thought, no, this is going to interfere. If I talk about this, it's just going to create a panic and become the focus rather than just one aspect of the whole picture. Many who might read this book and be helped by it, might be hurt instead. So I simply began deleting what I had written about this potential enemy.

Then, very late in the game, August, 2003, in large print, right on the cover of Reader's Digest, there it was in front of me again, mercury levels in fish, dental silver fillings (amalgams), and mercury in vaccines as possible enemies, causing disease. (27) Intuitive follower that I am, I took it as a sign and said, this is too important and it will be included. Besides if it's right there on the cover of Reader's Digest, disclosure already happened. Maybe I can simply raise awareness too and even caution people NOT to panic. Although, I would certainly think people eating an abundance of large fish, might want to research the topic themselves and see if the findings don't warrant a change in dietary intake, especially if their hair is falling out or if they're losing their memory or experiencing neuromuscular difficulties!

While reading the article I recalled the young woman who walked up to me at a writers' club meeting and told me that she had suffered many symptoms of disease, and when she got her amalgam fillings extracted, all of the symptoms went away. (I believe her by the way.) On the internet, many similar stories. Now, again, stories about people becoming disabled, frantically searching for the causes. Testing for mercury poisoning, registering high, then eliminating the fish from their diets and experiencing full recoveries.

Another flashback, one of the stories on the internet. One lady with ALS, how she heard about the mercury amalgam alleged toxicity, spent thousands to rid her mouth of the "poison" then nothing. Only one more devastating nightmare of false hope.

Very upsetting also, the one article by a seemingly credible resource claiming that some dentists might truly want to help, but others are telling everyone that walks into their office the very same thing. They *all* have mercury poisoning due to their amalgams.

In Reader's Digest, back to the article again, many credible people reporting stories about testing high for mercury poisoning, and recovering from heart-breaking illnesses after eliminating the fish from their diets. Even warnings from the EPA, stating the biggest risks are to those who eat large amounts of fish, the marine species and freshwater types. Also, the fact that "Advisories in the U.S. have been issued by 39 states and some tribes, warning against consumption of certain species of fish contamination with methylmercury."(28) However, that was in a report years ago. In the more current Reader's Digest article, it stated that even more states had issued warnings and apparently, women of child-bearing age or pregnant, and kids pose the gravest concerns for avoiding toxicity or ingesting only safe levels of fish intake.

All the researching I had done before, firm believers who link vaccines to autism due to (past use) of thimerosal, and its mercury content. The fact that mercury thermometers were discontinued. I began to wonder if mercury was like lead, another known hazard to our health.

My imagination even ran full speed ahead with the idea one day. I thought, what a fascinating Dean Koontz novel it would all make. Alzheimer's patients all over the world suddenly recover. They remember their family again. They realize where they are. They begin to walk a steady gait, talk and think clearly again. They all recover and end up on Oprah! Why? Those "silver fillings," the amalgams, they all went to the dentist and had them removed!

Flashbacks of asking one of the residents on the Alzheimer's unit to show me her teeth and when she did, I saw a lot of shiny silver, all in her teeth. Wanting, wishing that she could really be that lucky, that the damage done could be reversed because she's really a neat lady and because of something, one day she couldn't find her way home anymore or balance a checkbook or live in a real world or state of mind. Dean Koontz made it all sound so real with his super intelligent dog Einstein. Why couldn't it be real for all of the Alzheimer's-afflicted in the world? Extract all amalgam fillings, counterattack arthritis and blood vessel inflammation, and cure them all!

Then I remembered, just dreaming again. Yet, those people who got well, they aren't dreaming. Some people did recover, whether it was mercury filling extractions or elimination of fish. Potential does exist to prevent and counteract inflammation, prevent and counterattack immune-mediated diseases, and prevent and counterattack toxins which destroy our health. The less damage done, the better the recovery.

Thinking about the one evening out with the nephews and niece, stopping for some fast food before taking in a *Freaky Friday* hilarious movie. The picture in a newspaper of a young soldier returning home. That was the good news. The bad news? He now faced another challenge. The fight was on to counterattack a syndrome disease he obtained while serving his country. Now paralyzed and facing the unknown, he and his family frantically search for answers. I know in my heart that his recovery potential depends a lot on how much permanent damage is already done.

Nobody knows better than a hypersensitive how the body can be in such distress, over-reacting and causing havoc one minute, and how it can be completely functioning in a healthy manner the next. But those chances of recovery take a turn for the worst when permanent damage has occurred. Then, "optimal" health will be quite a different story.

Environmental stressors will challenge us the most I think, because they pose two dangers. Once aware of potential toxins and what they can do to us, not only do we have to worry about actual potential health hazards, we will immediately, consequently, also have to deal with the stress factor of fear, perceived danger. Similar to stress, there's good stress and there is bad stress. Well, awareness can be good and awareness can have adverse effects too.

To build mental and physical and spiritual forts of steel, we will have to be very careful to balance that beam between realistic fears and imagined or unfounded or unnecessary fears. To solve any puzzle, there are usually many pieces to be found. To truly make something whole and balanced in a healthy way, a holistic viewpoint is best.

Not only that, but adapting with all of our might is crucial to fight emotional terrorism of any kind. Scare tactics and real dangers can invade our senses to a dangerous level. Do we let those negative impacts win, or do we fight back, find a way to overcome the adversities all around us? Think of someone who has survived a concentration camp. If we envision ourselves as strong as these survivors and practice an iron will, perhaps we can free ourselves too of any emotional terrorism which is limiting our healing. While we might want to make it clear that a "concentration camp" of sorts really does exist, we may also be able to transcend its existence, if we keep working at it. Even be free one day, really free.

As sufferers of an illness, whether it's puzzling symptoms that come and go, pain which we cannot get rid of, cognitive declines, or more disabling neuromuscular signs and symptoms; validation is something we look for. Human beings are curious individuals and people know when something is not right, with subtle changes and with dramatic, more profound changes. When we become aware that something is wrong and we begin to fix it, hopefully there will be concerned people ready to help and eager to find valid, verifiable answers, especially a way to heal.

Awareness, education, a holistic perspective, reliable sources and people we can depend on; it's all so vital to our healthy existence.

By the way, the National Multiple Sclerosis Society, at this time, takes this stance with regard to the controversy about amalgam dental fillings and the implication of the proposed connection with the cause of MS. "There is no scientific evidence to connect the development of MS with dental fillings containing mercury. Although poisoning with heavy metals, such as mercury, lead, or manganese can damage the nervous system and produce symptoms such as tremor and weakness, the damage is inflicted in a different way and the course of the disorder is also different." (29)

MEDIC ALERT: Seems like I read that the removal process can also be potentially detrimental to health too. So again, caution is advised, and qualified medical and dental professionals should be contacted with regard to this matter.

B=BALANCE

Did you ever have trouble balancing a checkbook? Balancing work and family? Balancing work and play? It feels great when that out of whack feeling resumes a healthy balance, doesn't it? Terrible, when everything has gone haywire, right?

If we see our life as the balance beam and ourselves as the athlete trying to maintain balance while we "walk the line;" we can imagine the uneasy feeling of leaning to the right, jerking back toward the middle, leaning to the left, and again jerking back to the middle to regain our balance. Sometimes, even falling off the beam.

So many different things can get in our way to throw us off balance. If I had to pick one word, though, to represent the millions of factors that could create chaos, disorder, and imbalance, that term would be "stress." (Hans Selye wrote the book on that.)

Holistically speaking, (and for the purposes of this book and clarification, please note that I define holistic as looking at the whole picture and with relation to healthcare, treating the whole person, body, mind, and spirit), when someone is ill and seeks answers to heal, shouldn't that person consider each and every factor that might be contributing to causing disease?

I think in this modern day 21st century, most people agree that the mind and body are connected and interrelate to each other. If that's the case, whatever affects the mind, can affect the body, and whatever affects the body can surely affect the mind. It works both ways.

People who are sick and suffering are vulnerable. So while a victim of a disease is on a mission to remain a survivor of an affliction, rest assured, the books and remedies with a claim to help will be never-ending. Some might address the body, some books the mind, some both. Diet, nutrition, vitamin supplements, a myriad of "holistic" herbs and healing inventions, and a long list of alternative or "new Age" medicines and therapies might claim to offer solutions toward better health.

A balancing act will be difficult unless the right combination of effective therapeutic remedies are sought, discovered, and put into action. Whatever is out of balance must be addressed.

First and foremost, hopefully, the malfunctioning or over-reactive immune system can be counterattacked. It's a vicious cycle. Stress can affect our immune systems, and vice versa, over-reactive immune systems can create stress and affect our health and lives. What happens first will always be debated. It doesn't matter. What is essential, is to regain your balance as quickly as possible. There are probably many ways to counterattack from both angles of what is causing the imbalance. Again, however, I must emphasize, that many well-adjusted people and children, even pets are stricken with allergic or autoimmune related diseases. To approach an afflicted person, no matter what age, with the preconceptions that the individual is totally responsible for acquiring a disease, and absolutely able to make it quickly disappear with just the right magical remedy or alternative action, is not medically correct, in my book.

Talk about unbalanced. Though there are many positive results due to bold changes within a revolutionized healthcare delivery system, and many more options to turn to; we have simply gone too far. In my opinion, though there are many benefits, now we also have to worry about additional flaws in our changing healthcare delivery system. We're clear off the balance beam, knocked down on the mat, not knowing how to get up again. Why? Because a person can't walk into a medical office anymore with a real disease. It's all lifestyle, or stress, or this, or that or a problem that can be fixed within a week by some strange diet or vitamin or herbal supplement. (In some cases, maybe this is true. We need to stay open-minded, flexible enough to try options and especially eat more nutritiously. Unfortunately, sometimes it is not true, and critical diagnostic time is wasted for someone who may be very ill.)

So many of our diseases are certainly still related to unhealthy lifestyle choices. Yet, that doesn't mean that there are not diseases out there in the world to contend with. There always have been, and there probably always will be, given the dynamics of change.

Great wellness potential is possible though with many positive lifestyle changes and stress control ammunition. More than ever before, individuals are taking more responsibility for their own health. Many doctors, healthcare workers, and patients are becoming partners in a process toward betterment. All factors in a person's life are important to examine. Hopefully, a person can regain a healthier balance.

What parts of a life are out of balance, that's the key question to ask. To answer this question, a person might address the following areas of his or her life with regard to any positive or negative, strong or weak influences resulting from each: physical, mental, spiritual, educational, economical, environmental, occupational, familial, and societal. If I'm missing something, just fill in the blanks for your own life.

If you are sick, find a qualified, licensed doctor to help. Describe the symptoms, find the causes, and begin treatment. Then work on other areas of your life too.

Once examined, begin work. Try to get rid of the negative stressors, even if it means drastic changes are necessary. Your health will never improve if you don't. Of course, I don't want a parent to throw a kid away because the stress of being a parent sometimes has negative effects. But there probably is some way to readjust to make things less stressful, to make things more positive than negative. It might take a lot of work and time, but there are solutions out there, and within. The ability to adapt, change for the better, that will be the key. Quick answers too, such as divorce, or moving, often only delay actual stressors that show up again later, if the essential triggers to the problems were not addressed.

Smoking, negative relationships (without active healing going on), drug/alcohol abuse, and other negative addictions, they all have to go. Those you could throw out!

The quicker the better. Anything negatively affecting your life, you need to address, and make positive changes, so you can jump back on the balance beam and bounce around in a healthier fashion.

Change is never easy. It is however, inevitable, and sometimes extremely helpful.

So let's say you just spent six months changing for the better, got rid of many of the negative or unhealthy influences in your life and you are still very sick. Then, you must keep looking. The etiology of your disease has not been addressed adequately. Again, that unhealthy imbalance could be due to physical health, a disease process that is still plaguing you. There are many diseases of the body, mind, and spirit. You will have to keep searching. Hopefully, you will be lucky and find dedicated, genuinely concerned partners in health to help you along your journey away from disease, toward optimal health, and a sense of wholeness and peace.

A wonderful therapeutic aid in healing is the art of relaxation. I have a theory I'll share with you. The reason women are targeted 75% of the time with autoimmune related diseases? Hormonal factors play a definitive role, that's my opinion. Then there are the R and R factors. I don't think women have learned well enough, the healing remedies of rest and relaxation. I tend to be a tomboy. I ride a bike, I play tennis. Thank God I can still do both, although these days, for now, it's doubles tennis only. I wish I could play more cards and board games. On occasion, I still feel inclined to climb a tree or build a raft and float down the Mississippi River like Huck Finn. It's a busy world out there, at work, at home, and within. We are worthy of rest, relaxation, and play. Yet, I think the experts at this still seem to be primarily male. If we learn to play a little harder and rest and relax a little more, maybe that will help too.

May the positive forces of the world be with you.

C=COMMITMENT

I don't suppose you *ever* made a New Year's resolution and had trouble following through with that commitment. How many chances do we get in life, anyway, to make positive changes, to improve our health, to better ourselves?

The person who suffers a heart attack, even he or she can vow never to smoke again, to walk five miles a day, and to eat entirely different, healthier than ever before. But how long do those promises/convictions last? Forever? Or do they fade away into a forgotten territory of unconsciousness while the old self-destructive habits nestle right back into our everyday lives again?

Well, certain people with some diseases *have* to make changes. If not, it's only a matter of time before disability and or death will be the result of non-commitment. What if we're some where in the middle though? We're somewhat healthy or have healthy days, but we know we could achieve a higher level of well-being? We search for better health when we are sick, but do we always do what we can to stay our healthiest? Not if we participate in self-destructive habits. Not if we don't try to improve character defects. Not if we don't try and make changes in our lives that are necessary to enhance quality of life.

My current doctor, the one I was so lucky to find. He wrote a book titled *Powerful Partnering*. By the way, it's a book every patient and doctor willing to be a good partner in health should read. In one section Doctor Patchberg writes about growing in change. He writes: "Our cities, communities and daily lives are regularly confronted with untold trillions of changes. These changes demand an increasing awareness of how we must respond, react, adapt, and integrate. The changes we face are often chaotic, unplanned and disorderly. The natural world, by contrast, generally exhibits an amazing orderliness and predictability in its changes. Becoming change-masters in the civilized world involves a challenge to match the model of excellence found in the natural world." (30) He uses the life of a monarch butterfly as an example of "one of nature's most beautiful and inspiring" transitions.

I like this concept too. If we think of ourselves as mere eggs initially, fertilized and ready to grow, and as constantly changing and developing toward our fullest potential, I guess we could envision ourselves as beautiful butterflies at some point in our lives. However, I think many people stop short of their destined flights. They get stuck on the balance beam of life between stagnation and positive change. Sometimes, they even stumble backwards and give up trying to move forward again.

Abraham Maslow, ultimate believer in self-actualization, he wrote this as a positive mental health suggestion related to a person's troubled inner nature and possible adverse effects on health:

"If this essential core (inner nature) of the person is frustrated, denied or suppressed, sickness results, sometimes in obvious forms, sometimes in subtle and devious forms, sometimes immediately, sometimes later. These psychological illnesses include many more than those listed by the American Psychiatric Association. For instance, the character disorders and disturbances are now seen as far more important for the fate of the world than the classical neuroses or even the psychosis. From this point of view, new kinds of illnesses are dangerous, e.g., the diminished or stunted person, i.e., the loss of any of the defining characteristics of humanness, or personhood, the failure to grow to one's potential, valuelessness, etc." (31)

During sickness or even in good health, within the framework of our lives, if we are confronted with a choice, to change or not, do we accept the challenge or not? Do we stagnate or move forward? It's a simple question to ask. Certainly, though, it's much more complicated to answer, to develop a plan to change and stick with it.

While I would gladly participate on a debate team to challenge some diseases that the American Psychiatric Association might deem "psychological illnesses," especially if there are clear indications of an immune-mediated or hormonal basis; like Maslow, I am an ultimate believer in potential. Someone sick and suffering will need to believe in his or her potential to change, adapt, cope, improve whatever possible in a life facing the challenge of illness. Without the ability and power to do that, optimal well-being cannot be achieved.

Again, long-term commitment, how is it possible? Determination and resilience are about the best answers I can come up with. And perhaps, one of those bumper sticker professions I tote around on the back of my car. The fact that "A mind is like a parachute. It only works when it's open." If we, as struggling individuals are locked in fear by the terrorist immune-mediated biological wars within, anything else in our lives, or we are stunted by stagnating, unfulfilling self-destructive habits and attitudes; we will only be closing the doors of possibility toward wellness. If we are not flexible and open to hope and revitalized notions, in essence, to change and positive adaptation, imbalance will most probably be the result.

Did you ever hear the word habitude? Well, Dr. Patchberg defines it as such: "an attitude in process of becoming a solidified habit." I love his definition of healing too. "The process of managing and mobilizing all the powers possible in our reaction or response to circumstances, sickness, sorrow, stress, pain or brokenness, mostly by changing our attitudes so we can grow again." (32)

Since he's my very own doctor, I'm going to take advantage just one last time of his wisdom and with the Doc's permission, list some very good suggestions that may help with regard to that tough issue of commitment.

"Habitudes of change begin with the awareness we all have to change when we:

1. Become aware that something needs to be changed.
2. Understand/exert freedom to change.
3. Think about the possibilities for change.
4. Search our feelings as to whether we are ready for change, positive or negative.
5. Clearly define the changes we desire, beginning to imagine that the possibilities are a vivid reality.

6. Think about the purpose for change, and begin to plan specific goals.

7. Prioritize which changes need urgent attention and which can be put on the back burner.

8. Choose those changes with deep commitment.

9. Begin to act according to these priorities and choices.

10. Persist, hanging in there regardless of the opposition or difficulties.

11. Have confidence that, having done all the other micro-processes, we can become response-able to change, rather than merely reacting.

12. Positive change is the outcome-a habitude that occurs when we repetitively engage in these processes of growth. (33)

Life is like one of those mazes that you come across on the placemats at Pizza Hut. Growing up requires a great deal of changing, coping, adjusting. Sickness, tragedies that crash into our lives, eventual death of loved ones; there are so many times in our lives when we will need to adapt to some shift in reality. If we try our best to work our way through the mazes of events and circumstances and learn creative, healthy ways to endure; fewer roadblocks and obstacles will daunt or disable us.

Attitude, habitude, persistence, and commitment are all tools to counterattack stressors which create disharmony.

Be forever vigilant in facing your life in general as well as any immunological facts of life creating havoc. Commit to strive for your optimal health, and you just might achieve it.

Well wishes for your success.

Sometimes, people who deal with the problems of hypersensitivity or autoimmune disease will understandably feel like, "It's not fair. Why do I have to change or be so careful or have to worry about so many things other people don't? It's not fair when people smoke and drink and eat what they want and still can do so many things without getting sick."

I feel the same. To the point where I often jokingly say, "Heck with it, maybe I should just take up smoking and drinking, and maybe I'd feel a lot better."

Trouble is, I'd just get sick and have to recover. As a hypersensitive, I know there is already a lot working against me to cause havoc. Whatever I can do to prevent problems, and muster up all the positive advantages, that's what I need to work on. We need to build strong, resilient mental, physical, social, and spiritual defenses, a protective fortress of human determination and counteraction; otherwise the stoic weak links will be our worst enemies in the end.

Again, why some people must face more obstacles than others, it's a lifelong mystery.

To me though, there is nobody stronger or luckier than the physically and or mentally challenged individual who forges forward toward optimal functioning and well-being.

That dynamic process from sickness to optimal wellness, even if limitations exist, happens because of change. Awareness, balance, commitment and the willingness and determination to "adapt and adjust" as a local ALS survivor puts it, will help us all to live out our lives proudly and in a healthy fashion.

We are never alone in this noble effort. Our heroes, those who fought before us, and those who fight among us, are always nearby. The human spirit of commitment cannot be crushed, if we do not let it. Nothing can ever change that!

CHAPTER SIX

9-1-1: A Call for Help
and "The Emergency Is . . ."

EMS: 9-1-1. What is your emergency?

CALLER: Hypersensitive, self-attacking and malfunctioning immune systems.

EMS: Where is your location?

CALLER: All over the world, inside human bodies.

EMS: When did this happen, is it happening right now?

CALLER: It happens every day, every minute, and yes, it's happening within millions of people right now.

EMS: What is your name? Who's calling?

CALLER: My name? My name is not what counts. I'm just one of millions who endures hypersensitivity. I could be anyone, your significant other, your parent, your child, your neighbor, your teacher, trust me, someone you know is suffering or dying right now.

EMS: Let me switch you over to my supervisor to see what we can do.

CALLER: Thank you.

EMS: Hello, do you have a specific emergency?

CALLER: Yes, this is a MEDIC ALERT! Millions are suffering or becoming disabled or dying right now because of hypersensitivity, autoimmunity, even immunodeficiency. This is a call for help, for increased understanding regarding immune-mediated diseases/emergencies. Please help!

EMS: What can we do?

CALLER: Understand the problem. Tell your medics, doctors, nurses too. Please understand and help. Thank you!

CHAPTER SEVEN

Modern Day Healthcare:
PROMISES AND FLAWS

D id you ever wonder what the world, (perhaps your health and life) would be like if smoking, obesity, sedentary lifestyles, drug and alcohol abuse, other negative addictive habits, pollution, and social problems such as poverty and crime did not exist? In our wildest dreams, we *can* envision such a worthy, beautiful, safe, healthy existence and planet.

As an individual and a nurse, I have always believed in the power of preventive medicine. I, like many others, may not *always* practice it, but I certainly believe wholeheartedly in health promotion and the phenomenal ability to prevent many diseases. Also, the ability to manage others.

Yet, what is the definition of preventive medicine? Immunization comes to mind, sanitization and safety measures, stop-smoking and start exercising programs, the practice of stress reduction and relaxation. Nutritional improvement would also probably fall under the category of preventive medicine.

Addressing the topic abstractly, wouldn't a dose of love, kindness, humor, understanding and support, aide in health promotion and disease prevention too?

If I truly thought in terms of prevention, this book could be titled *Autoimmunity Prevention*. Personally, I would love to tell all hypersensitive and autoimmune-afflicted individuals to stop worrying, a preventive vaccine and or anecdotal vaccine or medication has just been discovered to cure all of our problems. Receive this injection and you will be protected and healed!

If counterattacking was still necessary at times, maybe it would come in the form of self-injections, such as insulin for diabetics. I'd pass out handy immunometers, and as soon as an abnormal level of hyperactivity or autoimmunity read high, an exact amount of anti-inflammatory or immunosuppressive anecdote would be self-administered. I guess the epinephrine emergency injection kit would be the closest we have to that, for allergic reactions anyway.

In the meantime, however, modern day healthcare is what we have at our fingertips. Is it better these days, or worse? In my opinion, we have come a long way, but we sure do have a long way to go, too.

Let me tell you a story. When I was in college, sitting around feeling inspired about the revolutionized holistic healthcare movement, knowing, from a former sick person's viewpoint, that dealing with all factors in a person's life is important to get well; I also often felt lost and bewildered. It had gotten far too complicated. That pendulum, it wasn't balanced at all. Suddenly much of the good that was apparent seemed fogged up and lost because of the negatives, cons and adverse extremes which would haunt an otherwise potentially revitalized, healing paradigm.

In class one day, I realized that there was no room any longer for any real diseases. Lifestyle, it's still true, so much can be prevented and changed for the better if self-destructive habits are deleted. But I remember too, how allergies and asthma were viewed, especially in psychology class, as psychosomatic illnesses. The professor, someone I truly admired by the way, spoke of the advantages of being sick. How the kid got to stay home, he or she was pampered, all of that. When I handed that same professor a copy of my autobiography, rough draft, which dealt with the history of a sick kid with two very real chronic diseases, allergies and asthma; I'll never forget his response.

"Well, let me know how it turns out." Dr. Siv responded. And he said it as monotone-like as he could.

It became stark clear to me. From his perspective, I didn't endure any real disease throughout my life. It was all in my head. There was no physiological basis for allergies and asthma. And I knew right then and there, that this attitude would carry over toward many other diseases and afflictions.

Holistic healthcare revolutionary thinking: "We can cure anything. There are no limitations. There are no real diseases. There are only people with problems. Once those problems are dealt with, the person will heal. Voila! No more disease." Yet, I wanted to explain to him, and other skeptics that I'd never understand how a two year old, allergic or lactose intolerant to milk is supposed to biofeedback his or her way out of the very unhealthy predicament. I just don't know how a person allergic to bee stings or peanuts or whatever is supposed to simply mentally "cure" his or her hypersensitive immune system.

Also, as a sick kid who grew up in a very lovable atmosphere, but an incredibly unhealthy smoky one; I can tell you this. I did not want to miss school. I did not want to fall behind. I did not want to be different. I did not have advantages because of my allergies and asthma. All I got was lost days, a poor education, and lots of grief while trying to breathe and grow up. TO MENTION, as I tried to run and play and participate, I always had to pay for it, usually with an asthma attack!

So is our modern healthcare system better or worse? More promise than flaws? Oh, I think the promise that it shows is remarkable. Unfortunately, the flaws are outrageously incredible, meaning hard to believe. I guess that's because vulnerable, sick, searching people do want to believe in the power of magic, and especially quick-fix cures.

No amount of health education pamphlets would have changed that professor's beliefs about allergies and asthma as psychologically-based illnesses. Any illness includes psychological aspects. Since we are human beings with minds; there is no denying that mental as well as physical health is important to examine. I love the holistic concept, to think of all factors involved. But just because a person with say for example, Parkinson's disease, develops some degree of depression due to the negative effects of the illness, and loss of physical abilities; it doesn't mean that the person caused the Parkinson's. Prior to the Parkinson's disease, that person may have been just fine, a fully functioning, upbeat person. (I can certainly think of one fine example of a person like this!)

And for the record, I know so many challenged individuals, with one disease or disability or another, and they are still optimal functioning, upbeat, inspiring people, despite their obstacles.

Well, the same is true for so many illnesses today. If a person complains of pain, of disabling symptoms that come and go, of chronic fatigue; that person may be distressed because of health problems, but that sure doesn't mean it's all in their head. Are we supposed to smile and fake being happy when we feel miserable? No, it's a normal reaction to be concerned and upset when we have symptoms that interfere with our health.

This is merely an opinion. But I think we are living in the day and age when autoimmunity and hypersensitivity are just as important as destructive lifestyles to consider when trying to prevent and treat modern day diseases. The best analogy I can think of is this: A person walks into an alternative treatment center. The complaints range from headaches, lots of pain, numbness, to some short-term memory loss. That patient begins an extremist fad diet, exercise program, and biofeedback.

If the person has a brain tumor that requires an immediate lifesaving operation, will any of that really help the situation or make it worse? Shouldn't the brain tumor be diagnosed and promptly attended to?

The same is true for hypersensitive and autoimmune related illnesses. Initially, diagnosis is crucial, then preventing, treating, and counterattacking the symptoms is essential.

So where does someone find preventive medicine, if stricken with these afflictions?

Well, take it from someone who knows. There's only one thing that comes to mind when chronic fatigue, or chronic pain, or flare-ups of systemic disability occurs; that thing is called survival. A nightmare begins. The only real measure of existence, soon becomes the pain and disability a stricken individual faces. Until at some turning point in time, answers begin to solve the agonizing mystery.

Hopefully, this happens *before* permanent damage occurs.

A patient, and a doctor, often a rheumatologist and a family physician try to end or ease the nightmare by evaluations, diagnostic tests, recommended treatment and solutions and especially by increasing health education awareness regarding the specific disease process occurring.

A plan of treatment is mapped out, supportive measures such as national or local organizations are contacted, a follow-up aftercare plan is outlined, and a sick individual is on his or her way to improved health, right?

Well, maybe. Remember though, autoimmune related diseases are some of the "most poorly understood and poorly recognized." Although the sequence of actions I just mentioned might happen, far too often, timely and costly detours are encountered.

Since symptoms come and go, and often the doctor cannot see what the person is talking about; complaining patients are not taken seriously, nor are the potentially disabling symptoms described. To make matters worse, patients often look healthy unless a flare-up is occurring at the time of an appointment.

If someone chooses to seek an alternative practitioner and unorthodox treatments, help may come sooner, but often, also, it may not. While alternative or integrative approaches may offer help to some, at times, unfortunately, disadvantages and flaws in the revolutionized healthcare treatment field exist.

Again, if autoimmunity or hypersensitivity is the root of the problem, then if not addressed, the cause continues to go untreated. Without counteraction, a healthier immunological equilibrium will not be attained.

Similar to a diabetic in need of insulin to balance out the blood sugar, those with hypersensitivity or autoimmune disease need to counterattack to balance out the immune system. Detours will only delay help. Also, damage can ensue if someone is not careful.

What if that diabetic decided to follow some well-intended but unqualified "nutritionist's" advice and began an unbalanced diet, out of whack with regard to adequate proportions of carbohydrates, protein and fat content. That diabetic may end up very ill due to a condition called ketosis. Ketosis is the accumulation in the body of ketone bodies and levels to acetone or diacetic acid in the urine. This results from the incomplete metabolism of fatty acids, generally from CHO deficiency or inadequate utilization and is commonly observed in starvation, high fat diets, pregnancy, and following ether anesthesia and most significantly in diabetes mellitus. (34)

The same kind of imbalance can happen with lupus sufferers. I read it (somewhere), that alfalfa sprouts can activate the immune system and increase inflammation in people with lupus due to an amino acid, l-canavanine. This is a good example of how one person's intended "healthy" food may actually be someone else's "sickness" food.

The same with food allergies and sensitivity. Maybe there are some very effective herbal or dietary remedies for rheumatoid arthritis. But if someone drinks a juice or tea that causes an allergy, it will only make matters worse and add one more piece to an already bewildering disease-related puzzle to solve.

I touched on the concept of quackery or fraudulent claims already. I'd like to delve even deeper into this fascinating, yet disheartening topic here.

However, if something really works for someone, I'd encourage you to keep right on doing what you're doing. So often, it will be trial and error that determines what works and what doesn't. If we are lucky enough to discover an anecdote, why on earth waste a counteractive wonder? I'm serious!

While I hate the idea of a vulnerable, sick person being taken advantage of, I also acknowledge the continued mysteries of the medicinal world.

Some of the most miraculous medicines known to humankind were probably discovered because some brave, sick individual decided to try a more natural substance than a man-made drug. For instance, a special tea containing the common foxglove herb, Digitalis, which is used for malfunctioning hearts. Seems like I read about this as a good example.

Preventive medicine should be just that, a drug or remedy that prevents illness or suffering. Counteractive medicine attacks a disease process and tries to reverse or destroy the pathology occurring. The goal is a restoration to optimal health.

Perhaps the most important balance beam a sick person will walk, is the one called medicine or healthcare management. A balancing act between orthodox and alternative options will play a crucial role in the healing process.

The thing to remember while trying to maintain balance on that beam is the fact that self-responsibility allows free will and determination to understand what works within the realms of orthodox and or alternative medicine.

On the road away from disability and death toward optimal health, nothing could be more critical than those first few steps taken with the help of an initial power of belief. Begin with a skeptical, doubtful attitude, and perhaps nothing will work.

So, I'd definitely advise a healthy first dose of hope and faith to be a high priority on a medicine list. However, as educated human beings, it doesn't hurt to be on the lookout for exploitive, false hope promises. Billions of dollars are spent every year on medicines and remedies that offer little more than false hope. I'm sure in some cases, a dose of hope related to whatever else was taken as medicine, was helpful to some degree. And given the sad, realistic state of affairs regarding an absolutely crazed, overused pharmacologically oriented society; with iotrogenic adverse effects backlashing on a steady basis all across America; we do indeed need other options. But false hope is just another temporary fix and sometimes medications don't always keep working.

In an affidavit filed by Doctor Aaron Primack, April 26, 2001, the doctor was asked by the Federal Trade Commission to provide an opinion regarding claims made by an herb and dietary supplemental supplier. The claims and hopes implied effective treatment and cures for many serious illnesses including AIDs, cancer, and Alzheimer's disease.

Here is the general consensus of what Dr. Primack concluded: Claims are based on "erroneous information and can cause patients to do themselves harm when thinking they can help themselves." Dr. Primack was especially concerned about the notion or advice that "patients forgo standard medical treatments in favor of purchasing its remedies because people suffering from cancer respond to surgery, chemotherapy and/or radiation treatment. They do not, however, respond to no treatment, which is what the suggested remedies amount to." I found it very interesting also about his concern for those with arthritis afflictions. Dr. Primack explained that "allopathic treatment of arthritis relieves the suffering and reverses much of the relentless inflammation. It would be a major regression for patients to forgo the use of these products in favor of treatments expounded in the defendant's books." (35)

Again, the balancing act of health education. Weigh the pros and cons of everything that comes your way. Beware, also, of scare tactics. Remember to balance realistic fears and over-exaggerated ones.

It's only natural though, that sick individuals would want to believe the claims and promises made by those selling allegedly magical curative products. Maybe some will work. Often a chronically ill person feels as if there is not that much to lose by trying something. If it works, great. If not though, I would think, at the very least, a quick refund and apology would be offered in return for false hope.

I hear those claims all the time, "Money back guarantee." Well, sometimes that only pertains to unopened merchandise. How are you going to know if something works or not, if you don't try it?

There is a thing called objectivity. In sickness, that thing loses all meaning and value. That's understandable. Good health is a precious thing to lose. People are willing to try anything to get it back.

That loss of objectivity is not so appropriate though, with relation to consumer's rights. As Americans, we have the right to be protected from fraudulent peddlers and charlatans who make money off of sick people.

I'm sure there is a difference between someone who truly wants to help and believes in the product or technique being sold and someone who knows better and is just out to make money. Even then, maybe they're playing that "placebo effect" wild card, knowing that some people do heal when they are handed medicine and a promise that it will heal the sick. Tell someone that "this will make you feel better," and there is always that possibility.

Yet, common sense can explain away these peddlers and practitioners. Are they around when things fail? Usually not. Fragmented healthcare with no follow through, it's just another flaw often present in both paradigms of healthcare, orthodox and alternative.

A healthcare revolution did occur and continues. Many positive changes have evolved. However, negative changes are also everywhere, including the internet, where some of the smartest charlatans are managing to get rich quick.

Those with truly humanitarian concerns boldly hanging out on the limbs of transition while fighting selfish or fraudulent interests need support and congratulations.

A different kind of flawed, detriment to our health system is underway, however. And if the flaws, kinks, and bad guys are not brought under a microscope of value, discovered for their true motives, and counterattacked; too many afflicted individuals will be sidetracked, detoured toward false hope; and in serious cases, disability and or death may be the end result.

How could any selfish interest be worth that? The thing is, there will always be people who care more about money than anything else. This always causes problems and makes it more difficult to get to the truth of matters.

If we as individuals and healthcare givers become complacent with relation to autoimmunity, hypersensitivity, disabling and deadly diseases, and the flaws within a revolutionized health movement; we will only become weaker as individuals and a nation. No longer a strong America with healthy Americans, we will suffer, and witness needless crippling and death. This immunological war of terrorism, we fight here in our own country. Not only that, but we fight each other. If we need to fight a war, shouldn't the enemies be foreigners, not fellow Americans?

We must all counterattack now! Like Richard Bach's fictitious soaring, adventurous bird Jonathan Livingston Seagull, we need to fly upward, toward our highest potential, not downward, descending into unnecessary sickness and death.

Preventive medicine is within our grasp. We just need to reach out and utilize it. Awareness, balance, commitment, that's where the real hope will be secure and long lasting.

In the meantime, health education should be at the top of our list of studies, even in grade school, and ongoing, not buried somewhere, only to be dug up later in life, as a health crisis strikes. That's why we are so gullible, because we lack health education and we are firm believers in quick, easy fixes. Well, patching up things helps for a little while, but not for long.

When sickness comes, we need to be able to find our way back to optimal health. Many physicians, coordinating healthcare professionals, and people who seek help are changing the way we combat disease. Partnerships and supportive teams are formed, and in combination with self-responsibility and self-capability of what a person can do for him or herself, and what others can provide; people are healing.

Prevention, of course, would be ideal with relation to hypersensitive and autoimmune related diseases. Well, researchers are working on that. I'd like to thank each and every one of them, past, present, and future. Thank you for caring, for understanding that something within the immune system went haywire, and for working hard to fix it.

In the meantime, we can learn about hypersensitivity and autoimmunity and educate others. We can in essence, prevent senseless disability and death, and promote and foster wellness. This is not a far away dream.

No, this is the revitalized revolutionary modern day world of healing medicine. May we all travel together toward the actualized potential of preventive medicine.

While we're traveling, we need places to go and doctors to help, clinics and doctors besides rheumatologists who are more accessible. Diagnostic screening centers specifically related to over-reactive and autoimmune diseases are crucial, especially for maladies so often misdiagnosed or poorly recognized or misunderstood such as: multiple sclerosis, lupus, fibromyalgia, chronic fatigue syndrome, ankylosing spondylitis, myasthenis gravis, rheumatoid arthritis, and other autoimmune diseases. Allergies and asthma too.

Also, screening for post-bacterial and viral infections is critical, as well as current bacterial and/or viral enemies that might be lurking about within the body, which keeps the immune system working overtime.

I just recently read a press release in Today@UCI, dated 7/19/03 that was very interesting. It deals with "a research team at the University of California Irvine's College of Medicine and in Lyon France, how the discovery was made of "a virus in the spinal cords of victims of amyotrophic lateral sclerosis (ALS)" or commonly known as Lou Gehrig's disease. "The finding provides the best evidence to date of a possible viral cause of the disease. Many researchers have suspected a viral link to ALS, but in this study we were able to identify a virus known for nerve damage in the exact areas of the nervous system that are affected by this disease."(36) But the researchers admitted that, "research is continuing to determine whether the virus can be confirmed as the cause of the disease or whether it's a byproduct of a still-hidden cause of ALS." (37)

Autoimmune responses have also been suggested as one possible cause for motor neuron degeneration in ALS. Many factors and possible causes have been studied: the infectious culprits, environmental toxins, genetics or alterations of genetics with aging.

One of the major precursors of my illness was a strep throat infection. My brother was telling me one day on the phone about the author of Seabisquit, how she's dealt with chronic fatigue ever since a food poisoning episode years ago. I have run across a great deal of literature that hints at viral and bacterial causes for some of the autoimmune diseases and there are doctors who believe in treating rheumatoid arthritis with antibiotics. Allegedly, some "definitive scientific support for minocycline in the treatment of rheumatoid arthritis came with the MIRA trial in the United States. In this study, a double blind randomized placebo controlled trial was completed at six university centers involving 200 patients for nearly one year. With antibiotic therapy, 55% of the patients improved." (38)

Anti-inflammatories work wonders, but the class of drugs can have adverse effects, especially within the GI tract. So if antibiotics work, and actually counterattack the underlying cause of an illness, it certainly seems like a worthwhile strategy to try.

The best medicine I can think of though is understanding.

If someone sick can receive understanding, it can make all the difference in the world.

Again though, how does someone understand something invisible? If those of us afflicted walk into the doctor's office during a flare-up and have some signs and symptoms (or take that video with us with our hands and fingers all swollen up), we just might get lucky and receive that understanding we're yearning for. Otherwise, I'm afraid, misunderstanding and lack of credibility will continue to haunt us, wherever we go. Probably, especially in the workplace.

I could sit here all day and try and tell people what I've been through, especially before I found an anti-inflammatory that works and does not cause an allergic reaction. It all reminds me so much of what it was like growing up as an allergic/asthmatic. (Luckily allergy and asthma clinics are around for us these days.) Symptoms that come and go, symptoms people can't see, the interference with your life and work that almost makes everything impossible at times. You try to keep going, but because you do, people say, well you don't look sick to me or at least think it.

Well, now we need clinics for women (and the men and children who suffer these serious diseases) to walk into and receive understanding and swift, proper medical treatment. Not only that, but health education, research, and preventive measures. These diseases cripple and kill, and death does not come quickly. There is pain, lack of credibility and dignity, and one lost capability after another until a person is often worn down to a point wondering if there is anything at all that he or she can do to carry on. Yet preventive measures may save someone from permanent disability or eventual death.

I hate to play the gender card, but could it be that we need more females in power and money-controlling seats all around the world, especially in legislation where funds get allocated? For example, how many people know what lupus is? Many people have never even heard of it. Yet, people are familiar with AIDS, multiple sclerosis, cystic fibrosis, cerebral palsy, and sickle cell anemia, right? Well, lupus claims more victims in our dear country than many of these other diseases.

So, I, for one, as a health educator and someone who learned about the disease while sifting through materials to save my feet, hands, eyesight, cognitive function and memory, prevent a stroke and preserve quality of life, think it's time to spend some money on lupus, and all of the other autoimmune related diseases, as well as all of the immune system mediated diseases.

Inadequacies, flaws in healthcare often relate to insufficient funding. As we spend money on a war to fight terrorism, indeed a devil of an enemy; we should not forget the terrorist immunological wars that Americans fight every day of their lives. We need help to fight and win this war too, ideally, to prevent many unnecessary battles. Like terrorism, if we do not prevent and counterattack, many of us will not survive. Fight bravely, wisely, vow to never give up, unite and we will conquer. I hope to see us all marching together to the same drum, that of preventive medicine.

You know what else could make an impact on increased awareness with regard to autoimmune related diseases? Something I have coined as The AIRD (Autoimmune Related Disease) IMPACT program. The diagnostic and prevention plan could go something like this:

I=Implement a health education program and distribute pamphlets in every hospital, ER, doctor's office, women's health clinic and diagnostic center in the world.

M=Media exposure plans for outreach and educational purposes to prevent disability, death, and promote health for those with autoimmune diseases. Include facts, myths, fads, and fallacies.

P=Prioritize the needs of individuals with autoimmune related illnesses. Increased awareness, understanding, effective diagnosis, prevention, comprehensive treatment, and support are all essential to assist those in need of help.

A=Autoimmunity 101 should be taught in every college, medical and nursing school in the country, in the world.

C=Campaign for counteraction. Education should focus on ways to counterattack autoimmunity, especially in early stages of disease, because permanent disability may be prevented. Campaign for funding too, so research and health education can continue and be more effective.

T=Test the effectiveness of the AIRD IMPACT program and continue to revise and improve as needed and as much as possible.

I'd like to offer another option. Tell your stories. I just happen to self-publish books. A couple years back, I began a project called *HS-Hoosier Storybook*. It is an anthology of short stories written by Hoosiers. All I did was open a door of opportunity, asked for stories to be sent to me, and I would self-publish them. As read, so many stories touch the heart in tender places.

The same can be done with regard to autoimmunity. Send me your stories! Limit them to 1,000 words. I will edit and compile them, then publish. We can educate the world by sharing our stories and we can make a difference by creating a very important book entitled *AUTOIMMUNITY IMPACT ANTHOLOGY*. All profits will be donated to the American Autoimmune Related Disease Association. If the sick ever needed some "chicken soup" in order to feel a little better, it's us. (Send your stories to P.O. Box 42, Kewanna, Indiana, 46939, disk or typed.)

Just the other day, on the internet, I came across a documentary titled *Stories of Lupus*. (39) I'm sure the film helped tremendously to increase awareness regarding lupus.

Who knows, maybe it even saved someone from disability or death. Certainly, the important film helped many people feel less alone. I didn't know that Charles Kuralt endured lupus. In the fall of 1997, during national lupus awareness month, two women afflicted with lupus formed Mosaic Productions, uncovered and captured stories in a documentary with the intent to offer hope, healing, and greater understanding regarding autoimmunity and lupus.

That's what it takes to prevent tragedies, to prevent unnecessary suffering with regard to these diseases; health education and understanding.

Often a major flaw in modern day healthcare is inaction or the lack of health education. Major promise lies in action and counteraction. It's up to all of us to promise to do our best, all of us.

Many articles I read criticized health and disease agencies for not doing their jobs, for not spending enough money on research and discovering effective treatments for the categorical autoimmune afflictions and fibromyalgia (which may or may not include a definitive autoimmune causative factor).

However, I like to accentuate much of the positive facts that I read, and I did see where The National Institute of Health did develop a plan to counterattack. On January 10th, 2003, it was announced that the NIH "has released a plan to fight autoimmune diseases, a collection of disorders that affect an estimated 14 to 22 million Americans. Highlights of the plan include the following: studies to determine the burden of autoimmunity, the causes, clinical research centers for the purposes of diagnosis, treatment and prevention. Also, training, education, and information for those in the medical field and the general public will be made available utilizing the internet and ongoing public education campaigns." (40)

As I near the completion of this book, I'm trying to come up with the one most important factor with regard to understanding these diseases. The one thing that might help an afflicted person the most, and offer the hope and promise necessary for an improved quality of life. You know what I think? I think that one word sums it up. Here it is, four little letters. R-E-A-L.

To the medical profession, to the researchers, to family, friends, and the general public: These disabling, dehumanizing diseases afflicting millions are REAL. When we walk through the door and describe our symptoms, please understand that we're not making this stuff up. Our pain is real, the disabling symptoms that come and go are real, and the sooner health education relays that message and people understand this, then we can quit wasting time and put an end to useless detours and/or insults to our integrity. Yes, there will always be a small percentage of those who may take advantage of an illness or a few who no matter what, complain, complain, complain. There are some who constantly take advantage of one system or another which just makes it so much harder to believe the next person with REAL problems if some people fake it and lie and pretend sickness for ulterior motives.

However, when something is real and specific triggers are noted over and over again as a possible causative factor, seems to me it only makes sense to put two and two together and get to the bottom of the problem. I remember something about PMS being conceived as all in woman's head too. Didn't a major medical association want to claim women being plagued once a month, mentally ill? Even though their symptoms came and went with every cyclic "event?" Yes, I think at first they did. That's what I read many years back in Dr. Dalton's book anyway. But I'm sure they have "come a long way," too. I'm sure hormonal factors are taken seriously these days. I certainly hope so.

The age of onset with regard to my first symptoms, my hands swelling up twice the size that they should have been, it was forty-eight, exactly when I was experiencing pre-menopausal symptoms.

I never did think like some victims, "Maybe I'm going crazy," or question my symptoms, if they were real or not, think maybe I was imagining or exaggerating things or that by some magic I somehow brought them on by myself. What I felt was real. Disabling symptoms came and went, (except for the thoracic chest pain, it mostly stayed, for over a year!) but as an allergic and asthmatic, I was always used to that sort of thing. One minute disabled, the next just as happy and healthy as a lark, always grateful that the symptoms were reversible. Always so lucky.

Talk about promises. I promised myself that I would warn others, that's if I made it! I keep telling my doctor, "Dr. Patchberg, I don't know how I lived with that burning pain in my chest for so many months. I just don't know how I kept going."

I will say this with regard to psychological approaches to medicine, the body-mind cognitive approach. Everything I learned, in growing up, in college, in reading, it all helps to increase understanding and offer more options to try. When pain or illness takes over, it's tough to survive it. Every cognitive/relaxation technique I ever came across did help. It all helps. But it's not enough. Sometimes the treatment of diseases needs more than will power. It's called medicine. The effective treatment for over-reactive immune systems includes immunosuppressive and/or inflammatory meds. (For fibromyalgia, we're all still searching for the best preventive and counteractive meds for this agonizing affliction, although exercise might be at the top of the list.)

I'm so much healthier now, not cured, but better. Scars from this health crisis war do exist. Oh, you'd have to look closely, perhaps even virtually wear my hands and feet for a while, and my memory banks, but there are scars. Also, my left hand and arm, it's not the same. My left foot, not the same. My right arm, not the same. All of these body parts are changed. I think forever.

Like I said, I feel compelled to warn others. So from my all too real experience to you, someone who might be suffering, or someone who might be trying to understand these illnesses, so you can help; I promise you that if you understand that it is all real, you can quickly move forward toward healing.

Move speedily away from flawed thinking and interventions and swiftly toward the promise of optimal health. My hopes and prayers are with you.

While we're still talking about the hopes, promises and flaws of modern healthcare, let me address one more issue. While talking on the phone one day to a representative from the American Lupus Foundation, he made the statement that there is so much we still don't understand about Lupus.

Yet, to me, it seems like teaching people to understand that lupus is an immune disorder, this feat alone must be very helpful. Awareness and understanding are not cures, but may provide great medicinal effects to a curious mind, especially one in search of healing.

The why of it all. This is what we so often need to know. Why does the sunlight cause a problem? Why does physical activity, temperature extremes of hot and cold, emotional stress (good or bad) cause symptoms to flare? Why? This is what we want to know, crave to understand and what we want others to be aware of too.

Here is why, that "common thread." It's called over-reaction. Think of a person with a normal immune system. He or she gets stung by a bee. No problem, maybe a tiny red dot, a little itching. Now, let that bee sting someone hypersensitive to bee stings. The immune system goes haywire and pretty soon, if not brought under control, in most severe cases, anaphylactic shock, which can be fatal, can occur.

The same kind of thing happens over and over with autoimmune and hypersensitive afflicted individuals. Immune systems over-react to things, sunlight, temperatures, any kind of stressors, and physical activity. Like someone with a good-working pancreas and supply of insulin, blood sugar homeostasis can be maintained without intervention.

Diabetics, however, do not possess those healthy balancing capabilities. If hypersensitivity and autoimmunity were understood, people would know that our immune system does not work correctly or possess that healthy balancing capability, thus it cannot maintain immunological homeostasis.

To be understood, what a wonderful feeling.

And that other big "mystery?" We may not know all the answers yet to the puzzle regarding the gender disparity issue regarding autoimmune afflictions. However, there is one simple, definitive answer why women are so often the unlucky ones. Until this flaw in modern health care is understood, ignoring the hormonal factor, preventive and counteractive medicine will not reach its ultimate healing potential. This is strictly intuitive knowledge I'm sharing, but here goes. There are hormones that have the capacity to suppress or counterattack the adverse effects of a hypersensitive or malfunctioning immune system and inflammation. When those hormones are insufficient or defective, a person does not possess the necessary physiological ammunition to counterattack as reactions occur.

If, by chance, intuitive knowledge and veteran experience about a matter is not very convincing, then try this. I found it in my handy IN FOCUS AARDA newsletter.

Excerpted from "Sex differences in Autoimmunity," a Doctor Caroline C. Whitacre, Ohio State University, College of Medicine and Public Health, Nature Immunology, volume 2, number 9, September 2001. The doctor writes: "The increased prevalence of autoimmune disease in women, the sexual dimorphism of the immune response, and the modulatory effects of sex steroids on immune function in vitro have focused attention on the role of these hormones, mainly estrogen, progesterone, and testosterone, as primary mediators of the sex differences. High among research priorities in the area of sex differences is determination of the mechanisms by which these primary sex hormones, including estriol, affect immune function." She goes on to explain how "both multiple sclerosis and rheumatoid arthritis, disease activity decreases throughout pregnancy, but most profoundly during the third trimester when estrogen and progesterone concentrations are highest." Flares of disease activity, she states, occur postpartum, when "estrogen and progesterone concentrations fall." (41)

I'm with her, this doctor making such an important point to understand with relation to autoimmunity, hormones differ in males and females, so do the ratio rates of autoimmune related diseases between men and women, astoundingly.

One more extremely interesting concept before I go, just in case some radical researchers have really come across something. While checking to see if testosterone is actually immunosuppressive, I came across some information from a biologist named Dr. Braude. Dr. Braude says he's found some research that "questions the whole idea of immunosuppression and suggests that, instead of suppressing the immune system, testosterone and other steroids play a key role in what's called immunoredistribution. The redistribution hyposthesis predicts that when you are under stress the total number of immune cells in your body remains the same but are sent where they are most useful, to the skin to anticipate getting wounded and prevent infection." (42)

The doctor questions something I learned about long ago. He says, "You see it every day. If someone's stressed, they're likely to get sick. The simple interpretation is that the immune system is suppressed. It just doesn't make sense to suppress your immune system, even under stress." (43)

Of course not. Many of us are not getting sick because our immune system is suppressed. It's just the opposite. That's why hypersensitives often get sick. The immune system rushes to help, even against harmless substances or sunlight or physical stress. It doesn't know when to stop. If hormones are intact and can suppress, or redistribute, or counterattack, no problem, balance can be maintained. If not, then what? Hypersensitivity. Autoimmunity. It *would* make sense to try and suppress in cases of over-reaction and autoimmunity, right? That would mean the body is simply doing its thing, trying to adapt and cope.

It's all about balance, immunological equilibrium, whatever it takes. That's why I always say, don't go "boosting" *my* immune system. No, it's the opposite that I need, suppression; and that goes for millions of others too. Although, I guess the word "boost" could simply imply helping something to function better, in a healthier way.

CHAPTER EIGHT

Prelude to an Awareness
Fund-raiser

MADWAGON/WELL-WAGON

Not so sure about that name.
Think I'll have to make a quick change.
My new bike, my new ride.
Fell in love with it, so had to decide.
"Madwagon," my cross-country touring friend.
What a black beauty, I'll set a new trend!
From the Pacific coast to Floridian sands east,
Finally a dream come true, and then release.
Well-Wagon, Well-Wagon, carry me through.
Like pioneers rode, and settled in too.
Travelled endless days and starry nights,
Until destinations came clearly in sight.
Well-Wagon, Well-Wagon, cycle me home,
Where the heart beats strongest
And the healthiest roam.
September skies. Autumn winds.
Very soon, my adventure tour begins.
U.S.A. cross-country, American style.
Too bad, my Well-Wagon, there's no denial.
Not American made, but it chose me!
So coast to coast on my black beauty.
That's what it will be,
the ultimate dream-duty.

Isn't it funny the way dreams click into our hearts and minds? Some we pursue, others we just kind of set aside or forget about altogether.

A couple years ago, I attended the Midwest Writers Workshop in Muncie, Indiana. So many creative people inspired me.

One particular speaker, Diana Guthrie, an author of children's books, told her story about the five mile strolls she took on the sidewalks and streets all across the U.S.A. Of course she spoke about writing books for kids too, but I was more interested in the journey that she had experienced at age fifty-five.

I spoke with her later that morning and shared a dream of mine I had been contemplating. I said, "I'm thinking about traveling cross country on a bicycle to celebrate my fiftieth birthday." I'm sure my sanity probably came into question as I blurted out my secret ambition, but I figured, heck, she'd understand because of all that walking she did.

A few weeks later, I was home again, not dreaming about cross country bicycle touring, but just beginning the health crisis I have shared in this book. Like a sneaky, merciless sniper, the disabling attacks shot holes into my dream, until I thought for sure my dream was as dead as dead can be.

All my dreams really, even my life, I truly thought it had great potential to come to an end at one exhaustive point. Not an unfulfilled end. I always wanted my epitaph to say: If I should die before I wake, shed no tears for my sake, for I have truly lived." That, and if I died prematurely, I reminded my family to carve "car trouble" as a partial cause of death on my tombstone.

To be a chronic asthmatic, to learn how to be well and be able to participate in all the wonders of the world. When someone recovers greatly from an illness, every day thereafter is always just that, another extra day to enjoy. I'm one of the lucky ones. I escaped the ghetto of sickness and bathed in the sunny Land of Wellness. When fleeting thoughts entered my head and heart that it might finally all end, I accepted it and simply thanked God for all the special time I had been lucky enough to live here on earth.

There's always that "IF" factor though, when quality of life, even life seems to be in jeopardy. As I stared at Lance Armstrong's picture on my bedroom wall during the crucial days, I did what I had to do, balanced my thoughts between acceptance, and efforts to muster up enough energy to keep trying to get healthier, once again.

I thought to myself, March 16th, 2003, I've got a date with the west coast. And I'm not coming home until after I've walked on a sandy beach in Florida.

Well, here I sit at this very moment writing this chapter. Lance Armstrong's picture is still taped to my wall. He's on the move again, pedaling his heart away this summer. The champ ran into a little trouble the other day though, ran out of water, I read, but he persevered, of course. (I'll have to try hard not to do that!)

Me? I didn't make it to the coast on my birthday, March 16th, 2003. Too sick still. If I had tried, there was no doubt in my mind that by the second day, all I would be touring was a hospital full of doctors and nurses. It took me until April of 2003 to realize that the pain in my upper, outer left chest area might keep staying away for longer periods of time and I might keep healing, and getting even stronger. I thought I would have to live with it constantly for the rest of my life.

Mostly, as I continued to improve, it only seemed fair that since the dream of a coast to coast bicycle tour had played a part in enabling me to hang onto my fighting spirit, I should repay the favor, and if at all possible, keep the dream alive.

So that's just what I am planning to do. Dream and cycle on! While I'm sharing a big dream with you, let me share some smaller ones I had over and over again about a year ago. I dreamed of being able to use my fingers and hands without excruciating pain, to walk without pain too. During the many months that I locked the doors at work with the small allen wrench turnkey, that was a dream come true, a small miracle. To spend minutes, hours, days without that burning pain in my chest, that's an even bigger wish granted. And when I plant my feet firmly on the ground in San Diego, California in September, 2003 with my black beauty of a bike right next to me and get ready to ride; that, my dear readers, and fellow hypersensitive and autoimmune prone companions, will be an outrageously huge, fantastic miracle. I can't wait for the moment, to breathe in the reality that I made it. That I'm really here, and healthier than I ever thought I would be able to return to. Thank you God, from the center of my soul. Why me? Why am I so lucky? I don't know why, but thank you.

Now, for those who want to ride along with me, please get ready to "saddle in." Fellow hyper and autoimmune victims and survivors, are you there? Healthcare professionals, family, friends, researchers, Virginia, from the AARDA, are you there? It all starts here. Let's ride.

Montel, are you nearby? I don't see your camera crew. Maybe we're going to meet up further down the road. I really didn't want to get your attention too early anyway, too stressful to this over-reactive immune system of mine. Need to get things started first, it's easier that way. But hey, whatever media shows up, I'll welcome you. Please spread the news. Autoimmune and hypersensitive attacks cause horrendous suffering. It's time to COUNTERATTACK! Everyone can help by buying my book AND sending at least one dollar to the **American Autoimmune Related Diseases Association at: 22100 Gratiot Avenue, East Detroit, Michigan 48021-2227.** (Whenever you see this book or hear about it, that would be a perfect time to donate.)

Annette Funicello, seems like you were one of the first well-known people in the news that came forward and began to share your illness, MS, and educate us on the disease. By the way, is Frankie Avalon still around? I have this vision of all of us, you, Frankie, so he could sing at the event, and the entire population of people stricken with immune system related diseases gathering at St. Augustine's in Florida to enjoy a beach party/fund-raiser someday. We could call it a "Back to the Beach" bash! What do you think? Hey, maybe the rest of the Mouseketeers could make it too! Wouldn't that be fun! I'd love for you and Montel to meet my friend Anne. (Of course my cycling comrades are invited too!)

I just looked up Frankie on the net, and sure enough, he's still singing. (Happy birthday Mr. Avalon, I see your birthday is September 18th, the same as my mom's and the day I get ready to ride.) What do you think? Wouldn't that be fun? And for an exceptionally good cause too.

Tina Wesson, Kellie Martin, even Ken Wales, are you there? Spread the word. Remember, you helped to start all of this! Kellie, don't forget all of those actors in ER that you worked alongside of for a while. Here's their chance to really play doctor and nurse.

Oprah, are you there? If ever there was a women's health issue, here it is, autoimmunity. I've been sending you my books for years. Hope you paid attention when this one showed up in your mail.

Other celebrities, well-known people, and American and other worldly citizens, are you ready to help? Here's your chance. President Bush, your mother and father both are afflicted with Grave's disease, autoimmunity of the thyroid gland. Gail Devers (former Olympic athlete) and Carla Overbeck (former U.S. Soccer team captain), also Grave's disease survivors, can you help? Kim Alexis, survivor of Hashimoto's disease, passionate advocate for women's health, we need your help too!

Teri Garr, I understand you have MS. How are you managing? Gloria Estefan, your father, another afflicted loved one with multiple sclerosis. As loved ones are affected, so are we all, aren't we? J.K. Rowling, seems like I read one of your family members is in this afflicted boat too.

Wayne Newton, I see where you helped with a Gala Lupus fund-raiser already. Will you all help now? Mr. Bosley, from Happy Days, seems like you were helping out at a fund-raiser too. Howie, from the Backstreet Boys, I see your sister, sadly, died of lupus. Spread the word, autoimmunity is an etiology and category of disease.

To anyone who wants to help, buy my book, so profits can be there for organizations to help increase health education awareness regarding autoimmune related diseases. Also, please tell everyone you know to send, at least one dollar to AARDA. (More generous contributions, if you happen to have a lot of money. This is one of the best causes in the world. We can prevent permanent disability and/or death, also misunderstanding.)

National spokesperson for rheumatoid arthritis, Aida Turturro, (actress from The Soprano's), please do your thing and speak out.

To all the hypersensitive and/or autoimmune related disease sites on the internet, let's connect those links like never before! I'm dreaming big here folks, but I can't do it without all of you.

To all of the health organizations and teaching hospitals and research agencies and institutions, you are all probably already working extremely hard to ease our pain and suffering, and you can help here too by spreading the word, buying this book, and donating at least one dollar to AARDA. The major players in this field of medicine, especially, you know who you are, you can definitely be leaders in this unified effort to increase understanding and awareness with regard to some of the most devastating diseases of our current era.

Politicians, legislators, legal system staffers from court reporters to Supreme Court judges, please join in this effort to make a difference in the lives of millions.

A special plea to nursing homes across America, all over the world. Let's prevent some of the tragedy, delay some of the disease and heartbreak we see everyday in our work environment. There are current studies underway for heart disease, stokes and some neuromuscular disorders, to show that inflammation is a possible culprit. (Mr. Fox, are you there? We need your lucky charm! Bring your buddy

Mohammed too! There's a lot of inflammation that occurs following brain injuries.) Cancer and Alzheimer's too, right this very minute, more studies are being conducted to see if inflammation is a causative factor in all of these. If we can raise more money, we can increase research, raise awareness, and prevent inflammation and/or other specific triggers or counterattack early, with the very first signs. Preventive medicine for a change, not just acceptance, treating all of the devastating adverse effects, maintaining people who were not saved in time from a disease process that could have been stopped or delayed for years. Please contribute, and thanks for all that T.L.C. Sometimes it's the best medicine in the world, besides a cure.

Dr. Dobson, Focus on the Family, your radio show from sunny Denver, Colorado, you have helped so many people with your radio shows. Please send those T.L.C. waves charging and vibrating out all over the world. Sickness affects every part of our soul. Dr. Dobson and all churches, help us to counterattack and renew a healthy spirit! After all, miracles are in your line of work, aren't they? Henry and I have the antibody troops, the good guys, marching forward like never before, but we need that spiritual ammo too!

Talk show hosts, fellow Hoosier Mr. Letterman, I know how you get a kick out of someone sailing around the world or trying to climb a mountain and how you love it when it's someone from Indiana. **Well??** To those other goofy guys too, I don't know, do you see a story here?

Libraries, department stores, supermarkets, convenience stores, anything connected to a chain, and certainly schools, oh yes schools and colleges. Here's your chance to really teach something worthwhile and to join in a humanitarian effort to save victims from disability and death. How about a one day seminar or at least a class one day on autoimmune related diseases? Medical schools, of course, the highest ranking of all as far as importance. It all starts there.

Musicians, another powerful force in America. When people hurt, when the world aches during tragedies or disease, you come together to raise phenomenal amounts of money. If you or someone you know has been affected by an autoimmune related disease, please tune up your instruments, "band" together and play loudly and clearly, and do it for money. Send it to AARDA. We can start those health education and outreach programs earlier than ever with your help. Your voices, your music can work wonders to aid in healing the sick, even in preventing illness.

Women's clinics, lead the way. This is our medical problem 75% of the time. Diagnostic centers, please make sure you are educated with relation to autoimmune related diseases. You too can lead the way and work some exceptional preventive wonders just by listening, adequately diagnosing, providing guidance, and perhaps referring those in need to rheumatologists or neurologists or pain rehab centers whenever indicated.

To actors, actresses, it's a fact that celebrities bring more attention to matters, so if you'd like to step out into the spotlight and help this cause along, that would be fantastic. Julia Roberts, I know you have already advocated for funds regarding Rhett's syndrome. Did you know that some research does imply an autoimmune connection to autistic afflictions and Rhett's syndrome? And you're such a "pretty woman" too! It would be great to enlist your help.

Kids, are you out there? Anyone with an allowance or job, can you spare one dollar for a good cause? After all, kids have the biggest, kindest hearts in the world. I know you did your part and helped with our country's war on terrorism. If you'd like to join in, perhaps by the time you get older these disease will be well under control and much more understood so that hopefully you will be spared these immune-mediated nightmares.

Military forces, we need soldiers. From privates to the highest ranking officers, please support all of us here in America too as we combat hyper and (auto) immune system terrorism. Like any other war, we just can't let the bad guys win. Let's start the rescue mission. Captain Henry will lead the way!

Charitable organizations, millionaires who genuinely want to help and need a tax break. Spread the word.

Bookstores, look what you have the potential to do here. Just put the book on your shelves, most likely in the women's section, and leave it up to the women of the world to buy it and spread the word. You can help in the healing process because once we all unite and understand autoimmunity and hypersensitivity better, there will be a phenomenal dose of medicine known as support. That supportive message is as follows: Millions suffer from these afflictions, the adverse effects and the misunderstanding. That means, that no one person ever stands alone with these diseases. You are not alone.

Support and understanding is so extremely helpful. Support groups are out there. Literature is there for us. Doctors who understand these diseases are out there. We just have to keep looking sometimes, or educate a willing newcomer. A confession of mine. The reason I didn't attend a support group, mostly because I was always working when it was scheduled, or I was too tired to drive there. But down deep, I wanted to go at times and needed too. Yet, I didn't want to feel like a traitor once I got better, and that's where my heart, health, and life was headed. I don't know how to explain it, I guess writing is my best cathartic relief at times, yet it just can't be as comforting or real as a caring person, I wouldn't think. And to be honest, to be medically correct, I can only really claim to be afflicted with hypersensitivity. Autoantibodies, they may very well be roaming around inside of me, but if so, they have not been discovered.

Allergies, asthma, inflammation with use of body parts, yes, 6 out of 7 affirmative answers to one criteria questionnaire for rheumatoid arthritis, yes, 8 out of 10 (self-test for lupus) yes answers; much of it fits. And what is lupus? Did I cry "Wolf" when there was no wolf to beware of? That is the definition of lupus by the way, wolf. Around 1200 A.D., the most common theory was that the skin rash, like a wolf, seemed to eat away skin which had actually been bitten by a wolf. This referred moreso to discoid lupus with red skin ulcerations. Later, Sir William Osler, expanded the concept of systemic lupus erythematosus and recognized that some cases of S.L.E. occur without skin involvement but can involve the heart, lungs, joints, brain, kidneys, and stomach symptoms. (44)

All I know is I certainly had some werewolf of a disease chasing me, still do, and I've endured many vicious bites too! When a werewolf is lurking, a person needs to learn fast in order to prevent and counterattack quickly, as much as possible, to fight back. What is lupus, MS? What is rheumatoid arthritis? What is, polymyalgia rheumatica? All of these, which I have had symptoms of, relate to over-reactive attacks within the body, a condition that I was born with, one which I have encountered AND counterattacked all my life. Up until a few years ago, the attacks seemed more directed toward my asthmatic lungs and nasal passages. More recently, however, systemic attacks and neuromuscular affectations became the challenging aspects of concern and obstacles warranting counteraction, then learning the art of prevention.

I'd love to obtain more tests, but the rheumatologist appointment I was finally given is not until September 23. I'll be on the road by then. I called and tried to get an earlier one, but no such luck. Besides, my family doctor, he's fully capable of ordering any further tests. Mainly, I just want him to help me continue to counterattack, prevent flares, complications, and stay as healthy as possible.

Think I will ask for an MRI though, a cholesterol check before I leave and a few more antibody tests. I remember reading in Newsweek magazine, the July 14th, 2003 issue about Statin drugs. Coronary artery disease, multiple sclerosis, Alzheimer's, all of these diseases allegedly can be brought under better control, perhaps prevented, with the use of cholesterol lowering drugs. (45) Of course, exercise and eliminating destructive lifestyle habits should always be on the forefront of natural medicine, to see if additional medicine is even necessary.

Back to the enlistment of kind-hearted souls who want to help. I know I'm missing people out there, but I'm running out of time on this book. If I don't get it finished and into the printer within a week or so, it won't be at my side as I begin to travel when I start, or at least by October, for Lupus Awareness month. So, like the Academy Awards, just know that you are all included, if I forgot you. My family, friends, you've always been there for me. Just keep that endless love and support coming. To anyone and everyone who helps, eternal thanks.

Oh, and by the way, congratulations to Lance Armstrong once again. I'm sure everyone is wondering if he's going for number six. I'd better get busy and order that custom made t-shirt of mine. "Right behind you Lance! Hypersensitive and autoimmune disease SURVIVORS." Or, I can make it! A co-worker at work is a talented seamstress and she let me know all about these handy fabric markers. I can make up a bunch of t-shirts and sport whatever messages I want, including the name of this book and fund-raiser!

By the way, in the mail today, I just received a letter from guess who. You guessed it, Lance. So I need to join the American League of bicyclists, as requested. I already knew he believed in good causes, cancer funding, of course, at the top of his list.

What do you say champ, here's another good cause, right here. Feel free to direct all the kind hearts you've run into over the years toward this book and AARDA. I hope we can all pave the way and ride-on into the Land of Wellness.

There is one more important person that could sure help the cause. It's an amazing all-American publicist that lives out west. He says he loves my book, *Author Unknown*. I know, just give Montel a call. Once you know this book's going to sell, you can just jump right in. (Can you hear me talking to you Mr. Terrific publicist?) After all, this could be one of those fateful connections that was just meant to be. Have to pay attention to those.

Well, it's time to wrap this book up. I've got a date with the west coast soon. Lots of preparing to do. My legs are toned up, my back, it's hanging in there. (Trouble off and on since 1994. Broke one of the nursing code golden rules, worked without a back brace. So nurses and nurses' aides beware. A bad back will haunt you forever if injury is not avoided. Remember, preventive medicine!)

While I'm at it, I guess I broke another golden rule when I implied that I am one of the millions with systemic lupus. Nurses, we're not supposed to diagnose. The thing is, I take exception when it comes to my own health or disease.

Here's the most exciting news. As of this writing, that thoracic pain has stayed away longer than ever before, for weeks this time instead of days or one week. You know what, I'm knocking on wood right now, but I think I've beaten it. I really do. If so, that just means I'm a very lucky woman.

Oh, I got some of my latest test results back. Some abnormalties exist, though tests positive for RA and lupus have not been confirmed. Sedimentation rate is down from last time, so I seem to be managing/counteracting inflammation. White blood cells are low, BUN is high, A/G ratio is low, which refers to a decrease in albumin and an increase in globulin, and might signify the ongoing inflammatory response. Monocytes and Eosonophils are roaming around for certain, as well as some of those other crazed antibodies at times, I'm sure. Wish I could talk to Henry. He'd give me the holistic story, what's really going on inside of me, but he's busy educating the antibody troops regarding over-reaction, how it's so damaging and unnecessary and preparing them all for this educational tour.

Antistrep (ASO) titer showed within normal range. That was a relief, once again. I keep reading over and over again how a strep throat infection often starts something like this, a major health crisis.

While trying to be comprehensive, since this is supposed to be a holistic approach book, I wondered if I had to share this personal tidbit with you. I don't want to. Oh well, here goes. I think it might help some people, some people it won't. Just like me, it probably would have helped some, but I think all of it still would have happened. Unless maybe I could go back in time and NOT fall prey to a step throat infection and an allergic reaction to a medication, or if I could have been born without a hyper immune system.

Oral health. Mine's not the greatest. I got some work a few years back, sitting through hours of work, trying to help all my remaining teeth be in the best shape they could. But then everything came to a standstill. I realized many of them were too far gone. Yet I was not ready for the radical change of a whole mouthful of new teeth.

So given that other reading about how anything roaming around in the body, actual or perceived enemies, will probably be under attack, especially within hypersensitives, it could be that some of this is related to the dental factor. I'm sure it didn't help. Another thought. If I were one of the unlucky ones to be adversely affected by amalgams, it wouldn't help either to have it slowly dissolving away in my body. But there is a more obvious threat, those bacterial enemies. Wish I were a scientist and owned a laboratory. I'd test everything. I'd search until I found every possible contributory answer!

Some people will assuredly think, ah-ha, that's it, such a simple answer, concentrate on one factor. Well, feel free. However, the age, hormonal shifts, the strep throat infection, the allergic reaction to a medication; the constant reactions to physical stress; I think it was all going to happen and did. There is a thing called the whole picture.

Now, there's even one last health risk factor. When my doctor finds out about this high-exertion trip of mine, he's probably going to kill me. I'll leave a copy of this book for him before I go and reassure him that I'll be just fine, and of course call if I need to. Dr. Patchberg said he wanted me to exercise more, only following the Doc's orders. Oh and don't worry Doc, I adapted my handlebars, so I won't be stooped over straining my back. (I know I should tell him ahead, but I just can't. Too stressful, to witness his genuine concern and reservations about such an enervating challenge.)

I can't wait to meet my traveling companions, fellow adventurers who signed up for the trip with Adventure Cycling. Today I'll go buy my plane ticket to San Diego. Mostly I just keep cuddling with Holly and Sissy, poor things, I don't know what they'll do without their mom. Think I'll leave a taped message behind just for them, maybe that will help them to hang in there for two long months.

Well readers, hopefully supporters, see you on the road, as I'm traveling, in the fall, or later as I promote this book. If we don't make it to the beach for that fund-raising party this year, maybe at a later date. Take care and wish me luck.

For my writer friends, they might be wondering if a coast to coast bike tour book is on the agenda as I head out. Nope, not this time. This trip, it might be a fund-raiser and book promotion of sorts, but in essence, it is a vacation too, especially from that tough life as a writer. It's exhausting and keeps me trapped indoors often when I'd rather be out enjoying the fresh air. So if any of my riding partners are dreaming up a book, it's all yours. Just use a fictitious name for me though, okay, in case I get lost and end up in Mexico or crash and get all skinned up!

Now if you want to *publish* that book, let me know. I'll give you the low down on the easy does it self-publication modern day miracle called print on demand services.

There is a "but" to all of this though. It goes like this. But there is so much going on in my head and heart right now, and as I ride, I'm absolutely certain the sights and sounds and experience of it all will be spectacular and overwhelming. It's all got to find its way out of me and go somewhere. So I have decided to write only poetry during the trip. I'll title what will assuredly become a book, *Well-Wagon Train Poems, Recycled from Coast to Coast.* I'll close by sharing one poem already written. Signing off, farewell for now. Time to jump on the saddle and ride.

Let's get this bicycling Well-Wagon train rolling! Henry, all soldiers in this war, are you ready for battle? Hey, I just had an idea. For the afflicted troops fighting back, right along with us, let's simplify immune-mediated diseases even more. Let's identify, unite them all by tagging them with an I.D. For people afflicted with any one of the immune disorder diseases, we'll just hand out personal identification tags, an I.D., for Immune Disorder. What do you think? Forces unite, let's march! Counterattack!

I know war is never the answer, but those attacked must be defended! If ever I questioned myself about running off to battle, if I was truly meant to fight in this war against immunological terrorism; which I never did-then doubts would have assuredly disappeared last night. While searching through some boxes to find my red bicycling panniers from decades ago; I came across my little notebook journals that told all about the bike trip I took along the Pacific Coast back in 1979, almost half a lifetime ago. Travel date, the day I started to ride, the same exact date I begin to ride for this trip. I always knew it. This is just the rest of the story about a hypersensitive, Part II. There are millions of stories out there. My life is only one of them.

TOUGH TRAVEL DETOUR ENDS HERE

In the midst of
a summer and fall dream,
serfing on the waves of an idea.
Coasting now, on happy,
painless wheels of fortune
and able-joints in motion,
the nightmare detour signs
fade into a tough travel dead-end.
In the light, Hoosier sunrises.
Toward dusk, Hoosier sunsets.
Alas transformed into broader horizons,
U.S.A. skies, country ties with you.
Storms of danger resolved.
Healthy rainbows restored.
New road signs ahead.
San Diego, right this way.
St. Augustine, go east, that way.
Come travel with me.
See the sights,
hear the whispering winds,
feel the weather.
American Heartbeats of passion and beauty.
Sterling stars sporting magnificent backdrops
called life, from coast to coast.
Detour ends. Time to live the dream.
The reality road, paved smoothly.
Flashing signs spell poss-ability.
Green lights of harmonious destiny
cycling me home.
Home more than ever before.
Leader, lead the way.
Follow we will,
and wave good-bye to that
tough travel detour.
Time to ride *with* the wind.

CHAPTER NINE

TEN WORST CHRONOLOGICAL DISORDERS OF A HYPERSENSITIVE IMMUNE SYSTEM

10. As a young adult, I learned how to manage the allergies, asthma, to break free. Now once again, it felt like I had to live in a cautionary "bubble" and the only bubble I like is bubble gum.

9. Tennis is a game I love, but now cannot play with all my might. If I must live with this right arm, with its tingling sensations and swelling and look like Rod Laver, why can't I have his tennis game?

8. That burning sensation in upper/outer left chest area made me feel like walking into the ER many times, those other chest pains too, they were and still are occasionally scary. I don't like living scared, and hospitals are no fun. I never run into Ben Casey or Marcus Welby, or those cute doctors who play on the television show, ER. Most of the doctors are nice, but they all look at me funny because nothing shows abnormal and I look so "healthy." Say, don't they have any immunologists in the ER??

7. Waking up is always very painful at first. Instead of morning pain, it should be morning sunshine.

6. I still remember the boogey man. Disability, hands, fingers, wrists that didn't work, that made me scream in pain, aching feet that made life impossible. And pain, always the thoracic pain. It's always there, the bad memory, how life with chronic pain is often so utterly joyless, and life-limiting. I don't like thieves that steal joy. Wish I could see the boogey man so I could punch him in the nose!

5. Blood pressure. It's not fair. I never had troubles with it before all of this began. If I can't eat all the salty foods I want like pretzels and chips, and I exercise, and all that, why do I still have to worry about those blood vessels of mine? What's next, that nasty tasting salt

substitute. Hey, maybe I'll try that wonder drug, lipitor. I'd probably be allergic.

4. With the exception of major flare-ups, which I've been lucky enough to avoid lately, with the help of meds and preventive measures, my symptoms and problems are invisible to the human eye. That does kind of bother me at times.

3. This hypersensitivity, autoimmunity, and fibromyalgia stuff, it's all kind of unpredictable. I never know what's next or when. That too, is kind of scary. Preventing the unknown, that's kind of a hard task.

2. Like Michael J. Fox, often I just sit around and think how "lucky" I am. Lucky me, to understand hypersensitivity and survive it with such great quality of life, compared to many others, who may not have been so lucky. Unfortunately, I don't think people can see or comprehend how lucky I am. I don't think that would have been possible unless that (what could have happened scenario) would have happened. Talk about chronological DISorder. Let's just say I'm so lucky I'm not stroked out in a nursing home right now, or sitting in a motorized scooter, or sitting in an Alzheimer's unit in Indiana asking the same questions over and over again, or homeless because I just couldn't do it anymore, keep working at least part-time. So lucky too, because instead of constant joy, I could still be trying to survive constant pain. Lucky, lucky me. Though we may persevere when we are sick, nobody should underestimate the damage that an out of control immune-mediated disease can cause, nor should anyone underestimate the high level of recovery and healing that can occur once this medical problem is balanced, if helped in time, before permanent damage ensues, even after, to prevent further unnecessary heartbreak.

Another MEDIC ALERT before I move on to the number one chronological disorder. According to the Indiana Center for Multiple Sclerosis and Neuroimmunopathologic Disorders, in Indianapolis, Indiana, "If untreated, 30% of patients with multiple sclerosis will develop significant physical disability 25 years from onset. This prognosis is changing for patients with the advent of new treatments. Thus, preventing disease progression by using available medications is imperative." (46)

For the thousands every year, newly diagnosed and facing possible disability, I'm sure they would all like to know that everything possible is being done to avoid unnecessary disability and the maintenance of quality of life.

1. And the number one chronological disorder of this hypersensitive, malfunctioning immune system and nervous system of mine. The way my immune system acts like a traitor and attacks my own body, it's wrong and merciless. The way my nervous system enhances the pain response so it's magnified and I'm feeling pain more often and more intensely than I should be, it's all disorderly and chaotic and a shame people have to try and live like this, especially until some control is obtained. My immune system, my inner body, should not be my own worst enemy.

CHAPTER TEN

TEN BEST FURTHER SUGGESTIONS

10. STRIVE TO MAINTAIN A POSITIVE, HOPEFUL ATTITUDE, take a deep breath and know that help is on the way and especially persevere until you find it.

9. ADAPT: Find alternate ways of performing activities if necessary to prevent physical stress, prevent damage and complications. Be flexible and pace daily lifestyle routines.

8. DISCONTINUE unhealthy destructive lifestyle habits.

7. BED REST, favorite recliner chair rest or couch rest, *as needed*, will be one of the most important pathways to rejuvenation. *Think: rested body, rested mind and vice versa.*

6. EXERCISE or engage in physical therapy, occupational and recreational activities. Start gently, but after an okay from your doctor, proceed and keep moving.

5. PRACTICE HEALTHY NUTRITION: Remember some basics: less sugar, salt, unhealthy fat, and eat more whole grains, and fruits and vegetables. Counteract those free radicals!

4. FIND AND UTILIZE SUPPORT via family, friends, healthcare/ support professionals, spiritual leaders, and/or educational groups such as your local chapters of the Lupus Foundation of America, the Arthritis Foundation, etc.

3. PAIN MANAGEMENT: Study, understand pain and the fear of pain. Think of it as temporary. Develop a counteraction plan. Believe that you can overcome.

2. ALTERNATIVE THERAPIES AND STRESS MANAGEMENT: Keep an open mind. Be willing to try new things, as long as not harmful and okay with

your doctor. Offer TLC to yourself. Learn and practice the arts of holistic thinking (consideration of everything), and relaxation.

1. MANAGE your illness, then relax and live more naturally. Drift toward other preoccupations such as goals.

P.S.

**PAIN FREE
AND PAIN MANAGEMENT
WELL WISHES**

DEAR FELLOW CHRONIC PAIN SURVIVORS:

The late Emily Dickinson, gifted poet, wrote a poem about pain, something about how a person cannot remember when it started or if there was ever a pain-free time. Let's see if I can write a poem about pain too. Guess it would go like this:

"PAIN, a dominating monster,
An It, that claims all joy within.
From without, there may be no signs,
But from within, hearts and minds
Are crushed by a toll so heavily
That spirits may simply digress to dust,
To the nothingness that only aches and rusts.
To save ourselves, we must slay the monster,"
Or at least be smarter than It."

This letter to you is late in the game, because what often happens to me as a writer in the midst of a book project happened again. A few days later, and you probably wouldn't be reading this, yet it certainly would have been a crucial missing link.

While driving down the road, a radio show started talking to an author who had written a book about hypochondriasis or hypochondria, as we usually refer to the condition. It dawned on me, then and there, that fibromyalgia or the condition or syndrome which characterizes debilitating types of pain that cannot be detected with x-rays or other diagnostic tests is the perfect example of a modern day health crisis that many people deal with, try to endure, overcome, yet face being labeled a hypochondriac because there does not seem to be any proven reasons for the pain.

Even with systemic lupus, there may have been signs, symptoms, but the cause for some of the unnecessary deaths is because those afflicted may still "look" healthy. Yet, vital organs can be attacked, the pain worsens, bodily systems fail, and before a team of doctors even realizes the severity of the situation, it's too late, complications occur, and the patient sometimes dies.

Again, I agree with the tremendous adaptive capabilities that human beings possess. But this notion that we can simply overcome anything and everything, that all disease is our fault, that pain is all about emotional problems, or that women just like to complain, etc., it's all got to stop.

So often this type of thinking seems to pick on adults and ignores the fact that millions of kids suffer diseases too and fight courageous battles to be as healthy as possible.

What women, men, and children, who deal with chronic pain need is this: first, a diagnosis which could simply be labeled as chronic and/or intermittent pain, then this incredibly empathetic approach, understanding, and reaction as noted by The American Academy of Pain Medicine.

"Each physician bears the responsibility to evaluate and treat persistent pain as a serious medical condition. Principal treatment physicians must approach each patient with respect and urgency and provide appropriate and timely referrals to a Pain Medicine specialist when primary medical care has not been effective." (47)

The consensus statement further explains: "Like many illnesses that at one time were not well understood, pain and its many manifestations may be poorly treated and seriously underestimated. Inappropriately treated pain seriously compromises a patient's quality of life, causing emotional suffering and often leads to mood disorders, including depression and in rare cases, suicide." (48)

So as I was listening to the radio broadcast, I'm reflecting and realizing that I was a victim and now am a survivor of chronic pain. I could have easily remained derailed, if the pain had not gotten easier to deal with. I'm still so far behind on many goals, and the wounds are there, how pain took over and consumed my life and health. I'll never forget the nightmare. I remember at one low point I said, "Well, I guess I still have some quality of life." But actually, it didn't feel like it. I've always been an active person. I never did like to just sit around and talk and drink coffee. I like to go outside, walk, ride a bike, swim, even at work, I'm always busy. I just have to be active. So for me, the idea that I could not even sit still and be free of pain was absolutely devastating.

Whenever I thought about working on something, whenever I physically exerted myself, that pain in my upper, outer left chest area worsened and forced me to go right back to bed. I remember thinking, "This is not quality of life. I used to be able to feel so healthy." Yet, nobody could look at me and see anything wrong, except maybe the dark circles under my eyes, or the grimace of pain on my face as I did move about, or me holding my chest, or maybe if I lived with someone, they would have heard me crying a lot of times. But even back then, I hung onto whatever I could in my life. The pain was there but if I didn't go pick up my nephews and niece once in a while to go to a movie, or if I didn't walk the dogs or work at least a couple days a week, always enduring pain, never knowing how or if I could really get through the day; I would not have had anything.

I even showed up at the tennis courts once every two weeks on friday nights to socialize with some neat tennis enthusiasts and stimulate my natural endorphins for a few moments or hours of pain relief and specifically, to imagine myself healthy again. Had I not kept on going, my life to a dead-end, I knew there would be nothing left, nothing to come back to if I did ever get better.

I don't know how people live with pain. I don't know how I lived with it. And just the other day at work, again, the other kind of chest pains, the kind that make you wonder if a heart attack will be next. I just sat down and tried to relax and they went away. Times like that make me think of that polymyalgia rheumatica and temporal arteritis, inflammation of the artery stuff. Kind of scary because we can't look into our heart or arteries and see what shape they are in, not without a lot of technology and costly examination anyway.

I am so much healthier now, yet even that nagging, burning pain in my upper, outer left thoracic area and other symptoms still come at times. (Late entry: not since the beginning of August, 2003!) If I did not manage my hypersensitive immune system counteraction well, and wear wrist supports, and take the anti-inflammatories, I'm sure the flares would reoccur in my fingers, wrists, and feet. My left hand, wrist, arm, and both shoulder areas are still a nuisance and the most vulnerable at times. My neck, and the top of my back and shoulder areas too, if I work too long in one day typing this book, it all swells up, starts to push my head forward, then it's hard to hold my head up. Plus the whole chain of disordered events then puts extra stress on all of the rest of my back muscles. Knowing that I can get rid of it, the swelling, the burning chest pain, all of it at times, that I am one of the lucky ones; it makes all the difference. I wish everyone dealing with over-reactive afflictions and chronic pain, or intermittent serious pain, could be so lucky.

The best I can do though is try to offer hope, suggest a supportive family doctor, a pain specialist, and perhaps this: think of it as temporary and treatable. If that approach is taken, even if you've suffered for years; perhaps with understanding, effective rehabilitation your health and life can improve. For those who have lost so much, no, you may not be able to return to the life you had, but there are always new beginnings, especially if the level of pain can be lowered to a more tolerable degree of hurt.

To the doctors and pain specialists that are there for us, I'll say this. Thanks for being there. So often the search is on for years and we never find you. Just one important request. When we finally do find you, do us a favor. Before we do anything else and proceed to work hard once again, (this time with some help) on improving our health, can we just sit down and spend one hour, one hour to talk, express our feelings, and have you listen and acknowledge how devastating it has been to try and survive? Like any war or concentration camp survivor, our wounds may not be visible, but they exist. If still suffering in severe pain, we are not really even free yet.

I see from the internet that there is some type of petition regarding fibromyalgia, in support of disability payments for this affliction. While reading the histories of people who have suffered so miserably and lost so much, it's obvious that pain ruined their health and lives. Yet, what a disease to have, pain. Does anybody believe a victim of pain? I do.

My heart goes out to anyone afflicted with this disabling condition. I know exactly what it was like to live as a disabled person. Pain handicapped me, to the point of immobility at times. After those three days in bed, I was just lucky that the pain subsided, went down to a different level so I could function again. I was really lucky too, to find a job for a couple of months besides nursing. It got difficult after a while because it was a sit around and wait for the next client kind of job. I do a lot better and keep my mind functioning better when I'm busy. But for the time being, it was a lifesaver and what I needed, to slowly work myself back into the workforce and keep the pain in my chest from escalating. (So many neat people too! My co-workers were absolutely inspiring, and I even got a short story out of it!)

Well, back to the disability issue. I see the problems associated with granting disability payments to anyone walking into an office who claims to have pain. Pain there is no proof of, it's all just hear say. We all know how the system works. There would be abuse, overuse, then the ones who really need it would only become even less credible.

Nobody wants this disabling affliction, believe me. I'm sure I speak for all of us when I say, "We'd rather be pain-free and able to participate in life like anyone else." So many of the stories I read regarding chronic pain survivors, they all worked before, they had co-workers, provided skills, one was a police officer, several were nurses. They all WANTED to continue working. They even tried and suffered for years to work part-time. After a while though, the wear and tear, the pain at one point overwhelmed these victims, a productive working life faded into a memory. I detected hope over and over for another chance. But like I said, the first hour of medical help in these cases really should focus on one thing, an hour of TLC.

As far as being labeled as someone with yet another mysterious sounding hard to pronounce or spell modern day disease, I think I'd simply rather say, I deal with (or dealt with) chronic pain. (I also deal with the hypersensitivity, possibly autoimmune issues.) But, just like the hyperactive attention deficit deal with kids, fibromyalgia is probably going to be the next most diagnosed affliction in America. Remember, doctors have to label us, put down some type of disease or disorder if they want to write a prescription of any kind for a patient.

I reminded my doctor that one anti-inflammatory pill started the healing in my hands and feet and prednisone works so well for the flares. Often for polymyalgia rheumatica, doctors will actually administer prednisone, just to see if it is effective. If so, usually they think of the immune connection, and shy away from fibromyalgia. (49) So I told my doctor I thought he might be right about the chest area mysterious pain, how it comes and goes and doesn't show up on x-rays and how it seems that prednisone doesn't do the trick for it. Also, I explained to him, at one point, what else I had read, how many of these diseases seem to overlap.

What I do know is that pain is real. An adult knows what pain feels like. So when someone walks into an office and claims pain is interfering with a productive, active, healthy life, a doctor needs to believe the person and quickly begin the process of trying to help, even if it is simply a referral to a pain specialist.

Especially now, since just today, August 7, 2003, I came across some good news. It may just help provide some of that illusive proof pain sufferers have been needing all along. In a study supported in part by the National Fibromyalgia Research Association, the U.S. Army and the National Institute of Health, this remarkable research reported that, "researchers found it only took a mild pressure to produce self-reported feelings of pain in the fibromyalgia patients, while the control subjects tolerated the same pressure with little pain. In the patients, that same mild pressure also produced measurable brain responses in areas that process the sensation of pain. This new brain-scan study confirms scientifically what fibromyalgia patients have been telling a skeptical medical community for years, they're really in pain." (50)

These results were published in an issue of Arthritis and Rheumatism, the journal of the American College of Rheumatology. "The study offers the first objective method for corroborating what fibromyalgia patients report they feel, and what's going on in their brains at the precise moment they feel it." (51) Well, alas, maybe we can quit wasting time. Maybe now, those who suffer from agonizing, disabling pain can begin to receive the help they need, rather than sometimes being perceived as liars, lazy, and weak-minded attention seekers.

I cried as I read those stories about people who have been unlucky. Accidents, infections, illnesses, then pain happened one day in their lives, and from that day on, the devastating affliction became a relentless monster terrorizing its victims and halting dreams and goals, even destroying families. Like autoimmunity and hypersensitivity, the symptoms baffle, disrupt, cause havoc, maim, and kill. When pain happens, it's another affliction that must be counterattacked, again, as soon as possible, but with well-wishes that it's never too late.

Just like outreach health education and resources for autoimmunity and hypersensitivity; we need to do more for people afflicted with pain. Another crucial balance beam in healthcare will consist of the patient/doctor relationship. If doctors concede that pain is causing distress or disability and agree to help, and patients are also willing to work on ways of adaptation and coping, even if exact causes cannot be determined, other than some general centralized nervous system connection; then it could equate to a higher level of wellness and less pain-ridden days and moments for those suffering. Remember pain can be all consuming. Then, how much stress is created? And perception of deadly diseases due to all the unexplained pain, how damaging, how stressful is this?

If our central nervous system is simply enhanced, experiencing magnified pain levels for unnecessary reasons, then if we can think of the pain as harmless, not a threat to our inner body parts, just think of the pain as a harmless intensified nuisance, perhaps we can begin to control it, rather than eventually succumbing and enabling the pain to control our lives. Yet, believe me, I know how difficult it is to think about doing anything, let alone practicing a strong mental counteractive attitude, when pain is constantly causing major havoc.

I also cried when I came across the descriptive word, "burning," because that's how I had always described my thoracic pain, and I'd never heard anyone else use that word. One person did say it felt like "dry ice." Yet, I kept seeing it over and over. Nothing like "burning" with pain. What a way to live, or try to live.

Time to counterattack. Also, time to share the most important balance beam of all, mind and immunity, immunity and the mind. Immunity is defined in Tabor's Medical Dictionary on page I-8. It reads: "the state of being resistant to noxious agents or organisms due to previous exposure to the same agent or organism." (52) Noxious, by the way, means "injurious to health."

I don't think any vaccines exist to immunize us against pain and I do consider pain a noxious monster. Our best ammo here will be to receive expedient understanding help and support, and our powers to: adapt, learn, cope, change, persevere, to endure and hopefully overcome. Personally, I think checking into a pain rehab center might help. That's where you'll be understood!

Though I support helping the disabled financially, I'd like to see much of the money go toward prevention and healing instead.

Good luck with that most important balance beam, mind and immunity, immunity and the mind. No matter what afflictions, conflicts or crisis situations you encounter, counterattack! Kill the monsters of pain and adversity. Persevere and heal.

Pain-Free/Pain-Management Wishes and Best of Luck Always,

Anonymous GG, Author

RECOMMENDED READING

Recommended reading includes any literature or material that comes into your life regarding your obstacles. A journey toward wellness is often solitary and unique in many ways. A paradox exists. We share similarities, but uniqueness of body and soul are ever present. If you are willing to search, the answers will find you.

High priority on my list of most helpful, concise health education material, however, includes pamphlets from the various organizations that help those afflicted with the health obstacles of autoimmunity and/or hypersensitivity such as: the Lupus Foundation of America, The Arthritis Foundation, The Multiple Sclerosis Society, The National Association of Allergic and Infectious Diseases, The National Institute of Health, The National Institute of Arthritis and Musculoskeletal and Skin Diseases, and many more specifically related to particular afflictions.

In the free health education pamphlets provided, this is the best and quickest way toward understanding; and understanding leads to the prevention, treatment, and management of illness, sometimes even conquering it.

That book by Bach does come to mind again, *Jonathan Livingston Seagull*. Why? We all yearn to soar, to fly in the realm and calm blue skies of wellness and peace. If we free our hearts, we are all capable of such optimal wonder. We must be brave and never stop trying to fly higher and higher, for there is nothing more handicapped than a heart empty of hope.

For a few other reliable health education resources, try immunesupport.com on the net. The Harvard Newsletter, Mayo Clinic, and Consumer Reports on Health newsletters are available too. One cautionary note, as advised by a Lupus booklet, "Don't believe everything you read on the net." That's always good advice, check backgrounds and credentials. Although, sometimes somebody who has endured the same kind of crisis and survived, is our best teacher.

BIBLIOGRAPHY

1. American Autoimmune Disease Related Association. (AARDA) "Autoimmunity, A Major Women's Health Issue." Pamphlet.

2. Ibid. AARDA. Pamphlet directly above.

3. Meadows, Michelle. "Understanding Vaccine Safety: Immunization Remains Our Best Defense Against Deadly Disease," http:/www.fda.gov/fdac/features/2001/401_vacc.html June 4, 2003.

4. Ibid. Web site article directly above.

5. AARDA. "What Do These Diseases Have in Common? Autoimmunity." Pamphlet.

6. Ibid. Pamphlet directly above.

7. Rose, Noel R., M.D., Ph.D., "Autoimmunity-The Common Thread," http:/www.aarda.org/common-thread, AARDA InFocus Article, p.2.

8. Glasser, Ronald J., M.D., The Body is the Hero. New York: Bantam Books, 1979, p.96.

9. AARDA. "Autoimmunity, A Major Women's Health Issue." Pamphlet.

10. Ibid. AARDA. Pamphlet directly above.

11. Lucile Packard Children's Hospital, Stanford University Medical Center. "Pediatric Arthritis and Other Rheumatic Diseases." Statistics from CDC, Center for Disease Control and Prevention, NIAMS Diseases, NIH and the Arthritis Foundation. http://www.lpch.org/DiseaseHealthInfo/HealthLibrary/arthritis/stats.html. May 17, 2003.

12. Fackelman, Kathleen, USA TODAY. Study: "MS Cases on the Rise Among Children," August 19, 2003

13. Lupus.org, http://www.saclupus.org/oldfiles/what_is_lupus.html, August 19, 2003.

14. University of Washingon School of Medicine.
    Erythrocyte Sedimentation Rate (ESR).
    http://www.uwcme.org/courses/rheumatology/rheumla
    b/esr.html, August 19, 2003.

15. National Institute of Allergy and Infectious Diseases.
    NIH, Fact Sheet, January 2002.

16. RA Resources Rheumatoid Arthritis.
    http://www.Rheumatoid-arthritis-ra-treatment.com/
    contact-Rheumatoid-arthritis.htm, April 30, 2003.

17. The University of Chicago Magazine, Burton, William,
    "Death by Design," June 1996. http://magazine.
    uchicago.edu/9606/9606CellDeath.html.

18. Ibid. Article and web site directly above.

19. Glasser, Ronald J., M.D., The Body is the Hero. New
    York: Bantam Books, 1979, p.96.

20. National Institute of Arthritis and Musculoskeletal and
    Skin Diseases (NIAMS), Handout on Health:
    Rheumatoid Arthritis, http//ww.niams.nih.gov/
    hi/Topics/arthritis/rahandout.htm, August 19, 2003.

21. F.A.Q. Typing Injury, "Carpal Tunnel Syndrome,"
    http://www.tifaq.com/articles/carpal_tunnel_syndrome
    -sep98-well-connected.html, August 27, 2003.

22. Lupus Foundation of America, Northwest Indiana
    Chapter, Portage, In. Orientation to Lupus, second
    edition, April 2000, p.2. and AARDA. "Autoimmunity
    A Major Women's Health Issue," pamphlet, and
    NIAID, NIH, Fact Sheet, January 2002 and Active
    Biotech, www.activebiotech.com August 11, 2003.

23. ALS News. "Oxidative Stress A Marker for
    Alzheimer's," New York, Dec 04 (Reuters Health),
    http://alssurvivalguide.com/als_news/981204oxidative.
    htm, August 14, 2003.

24. Strand, Ray D., Dr., "Oxidative Stress,"
    http://www.nutritional-medicine.net/oxidative-
    stress.asp, August 14, 2003.

25. Ibid. Article directly above.

26. Ibid. Article, Strand, reference #24.

27. Ibid. Article, Stand, reference #24.

28. Jetter, Alexis, "How Safe is Your Food?" Reader's Digest, August 2003, pgs. 52-63.

29. Environmental Protection Agency. "Mercury Study Report to Congress: Overview," http://www.epa.gov/oar/mercover.html, August 28, 2003.

30. National Multiple Sclerosis Society. "Heavy Metals (Toxicology)," NMSS-Sourcebook, April 2003.

31. Hollenberg, E.L., Dr., Powerful Partnering, Fairfax,VA., Xulon Press, 2001, p.207.

32. Galvan, Gail M., Paycheck to Paycheck, Lincoln, NE, Iuniverse.com, Inc. 2000, p. 258.

33. Hollenberg, E.L., Dr., Powerful Partnering, Fairfax, VA., Xulon Press, 2001, p. 304.

34. Ibid. Reference directly above, p. 209.

35. Tabor's Medical Dictionary, F.A. Davis Company, Philadelphia, PA, 1973, p. K-6

36. http://www.quackwatch.org (See Affidavit of Dr. Aron Primack dated April 26, 2001.) Extracted August 20, 2001.

37. University of California, Irvine California, Today@UCI, "Virus Found in Nervous System of Lou Gehrig's Disease Victims,"http//www.today.uci.edu/ newsrelease_detail.asp?key=744, July 19, 2003.

38. Ibid. Reference directly above.

39. http://www.rheumatic.org/protocol.htm. "Physicians' Protocol for Using Antibiotics in Rheumatic Disease., August 27, 2003.

40. http://www.storiesoflupus.com. Extracted July 6, 2003.

41. Lupus Foundation of America. Lupus News, Volume 23, Number1, spring 2003, p.3.

42. AARDA. IN FOCUS, Volume 10, Number 4, December, 2002, p. 6.

43. Washington State University in St. Louis. Fitzpatrick, Tony, "Testosterone, Stress may not Suppress Immune System After All," http://news-info.wustl.edu/feature/1999/Sept99-testosterone.html. August 28, 2003.

44. Web article directly above.

45. Lupus Foundation of America, Northwest Indiana Chapter, Portage, In. Orientation to Lupus booklet, second edition, April 2000.

46. Noonan, David, "You Want Statins with That?" Newsweek, July 14, 2003, pgs. 50-56.

47. The Indiana Center for Multiple Sclerosis and Neuroimmunopathology Disorders. http://icmsnd.com.

48. American Academy of Pain. http://aapainmanage.org. Extracted July10, 2003.

49. Ibid. Reference directly above.

50. Immunesupport.com, http://www.immunesupport.com/fms_research/fma002.htm.

51. University of Michigan. Science Daily, "Fibromyalgia Pain isn't all in Patients' Heads, New Brain Study Finds, University of Michigan Health System, July 6, 2002, http://www.sciencedaily.com/020607073056.htm.

52. Ibid. Reference directly above.

53. Tabor's Medical Dictionary, F.A. Davis Company, Philadelphia, PA, 1973, p. I-8.

Made in the USA
Monee, IL
07 July 2026

56552245R00083